FOOD AND THE GUT REACTION
Intestinal Health through Diet

FOOD AND THE GUT REACTION
Intestinal Health through Diet

By
Elaine Gottschall
B.A., M.Sc.

The Kirkton Press
Kirkton, Ontario, Canada

Published by   The Kirkton Press
               R. R. #1
               Kirkton, Ont.
               N0K 1K0

Printed and bound in Canada

Orders for additional copies of this book may be sent to The Kirkton Press (an order form is
available on the last page of this book)

First Printing – June, 1987
7 8 9 10 11 12 WC 96 95 94 93 92

Canadian Cataloguing in Publication Data
Gottschall, Elaine Gloria
    Food and the Gut Reaction

Includes Index, Bibliography

ISBN 0-9692768-0-X

1. Intestines – Diseases – Diet therapy

RC860.G68   1987   6.3.2′8
C87-090019-6

OTABIND

Bound to stay open

Publisher's Note

Otabind (Ota-bind). This book has been bound
using the patented Otabind process. You can
open this book at any page, gently run your
finger down the spine, and the pages will lie flat.

ACKNOWLEDGEMENTS

In the research, writing, and publishing of this book I received moral, intellectual, and emotional support from many people. Among these, the following people stand out and to them goes my deepest appreciation:

Dr. Donald B. McMillan for his time, expertise, support, and friendship.

Patricia Wilson for her friendship and willingness to share her artistic talents by producing the illustrations.

Diane Jewkes for her patience and expertise in editing the manuscript.

Sue Brown, Callie Cesarini, Marge Moulton, Debbie Newsted, and Jane Sexsmith for their good humor and assistance in helping me execute the numerous revisions.

Valerie Tabone and Sandra Rule of the Department of Graphic Services (University of Western Ontario) for their cooperation and expertise in typesetting and artistic layout of the manuscript.

My husband, Herbert, for his unlimited patience, moral support, and continual prodding to ''write the book.''

My daughter, Judith Lynn Herod, and her friend, Tad Crohn, for their superb job of initial editing.

My daughter, Joan Beth Gottschall, for her continual encouragement.

IMPORTANT NOTICE TO THE READER:

This book contains a diet and nutritional information that, in the author's experience, has helped those who have followed it.

The author recognizes that the treatment of illness and the enhancement of health through diet should be supervised by a duly qualified physician. Readers should not engage in self-diagnosis and self-treatment. Consult your doctor before starting the regimen proposed here. This book will be particularly complemented by discussions with a physician who has a particular interest or training in nutrition.

The author and publisher do not assume medical or legal liability for the use or misuse of the information and regimen contained in this book.

The progress of science implies not only the accumulation of knowledge, but its organization, its unification, and this involves the periodic invention of new syntheses, coordinating existing knowledge, and of new hypotheses which give us methods of approaching the unknown.

George Sarton
Introduction to the *History of Science*

DEDICATION

This book is dedicated to the memory of
Dr. Sidney Valentine Haas
who first showed me the importance of understanding
the effect of food on the body.

TABLE OF CONTENTS

Chapter 1

PAST AND PRESENT

In 1951, after many years of clinical experience, Drs. Sidney V. and Merrill P. Haas published a book entitled *Management of Celiac Disease*. Directed to the medical community, the book documented the doctors' experiences in treating and curing hundreds of cases of celiac disease as well as cases of cystic fibrosis of the pancreas.[1] Their approach was dietary, and they used a well-balanced, normal diet that was highly specific as to the types of sugars and starches allowed. When patients followed this Specific Carbohydrate Diet for a minimum of one year, they were then able to return to a normal diet with complete and permanent disappearance of symptoms.

In 1958, we took our eight year old daughter to the Drs. Haas. Three years before she had been diagnosed by specialists as having incurable ulcerative colitis and her condition was deteriorating. The years of treatment with cortisone and sulfonamides, plus innumerable other medical approaches, had been unsuccessful and surgery seemed imminent. The Drs. Haas placed her on the Specific Carbohydrate Diet and within two years she was free of symptoms. She returned to eating normally after another few years, and has remained in excellent health for over twenty years.

Many students, friends, and others whom I have seen in my practice who were suffering from ulcerative colitis, Crohn's disease, celiac disease (not cured by a gluten-free diet), diverticulitis, and various types of chronic diarrhea have tried the Haas Diet and most of them are now free of their respective diseases. Some of the most dramatic and fastest recoveries have occurred in babies and young children with severe constipation and among children who, along with intestinal problems, had serious behavior problems. These included autistic-type hypoactivity as well as hyperactivity, often accompanied by severe and prolonged night terrors. Very often the behavior problems and night terrors cleared up within ten days after initiation of the Haas Specific Carbohydrate Diet. It is interesting to note that in June, 1985, the Schizophrenia Association of Great Britain launched a research project to investigate Dr. F. C. Dohan's research concerning a relationship between celiac disease and schizophrenia. The basis for this project is a strict grain-free, milk-free, low sugar diet, closely related to the Specific Carbohydrate Diet.[2,3]

Meanwhile in research laboratories throughout the world, investigators have been studying intestinal problems. Physicians and researchers have found that a special type of synthetic diet (chemical nutrients assembled in the laboratory) called an Elemental Diet shows great promise in the treatment of digestive and intestinal problems of all types. The malabsorption problem seen in cystic fibrosis of the pancreas as well as diarrhea which occurs after cancer chemotherapy have been overcome by the use of the synthetic Elemental Diet.[4,5] When used for patients with Crohn's disease, not only did symptoms disappear but children who had not grown properly for years showed dramatic weight and height gains while on the diet.[6] The level of sodium chloride in the perspiration (the sweat test which measures the severity of the condition) of children with cystic fibrosis of the pancreas decreased dramatically when these children were given the Elemental Diet.[7] Over six hundred scientific publications have appeared in medical journals in the 1970's and early 1980's testifying to the fact that this Elemental Diet is effective in correcting malabsorption and reversing the course of many intestinal disorders.[4] However, since the Elemental Diet is an artificial diet, usually administered via a stomach tube, it cannot be continued indefinitely. When it is discontinued, usually after six to eight weeks, improvement gradually decreases and symptoms usually return.

The common denominator underlying the effectiveness of both the natural Specific Carbohydrate Diet and the synthetic Elemental Diet is the type of carbohydrate which predominates. In the synthetic Elemental Diet, the principal carbohydrate is the single sugar, glucose, which, in biochemical circles, is called a monosaccharide (mono=one; saccharide=sugar) as contrasted with a two-sugar disaccharide such as sucrose (table sugar) or a many-sugar polysaccharide such as starch.

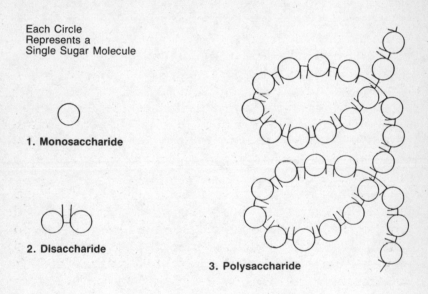

Each Circle
Represents a
Single Sugar Molecule

1. Monosaccharide

2. Disaccharide

3. Polysaccharide

Figure 1   Dietary carbohydrates

In the natural Specific Carbohydrate Diet, the carbohydrates are also predominantly single sugars - those found in fruit, honey, properly-made yoghurt, and certain vegetables. The many research reports indicating that the synthetic Elemental Diet is beneficial in intestinal diseases provide support for the Specific Carbohydrate Diet which can be used in the home.

Those who choose to follow the Specific Carbohydrate Diet need not feel deprived. Many of the delicious recipes in this book could easily be part of any gourmet cookbook. The fact that they are so appealing, however, in no way compromises the underlying scientific reasoning: the carbohydrates specified in the recipes are biochemically correct.

The Specific Carbohydrate Diet presented in this book is highly nutritious and well-balanced. It is safe and very likely to be effective in overcoming many lingering and vexing intestinal and digestive problems.

Chapter 2

SCIENTIFIC EVIDENCE RELATING TO DIET

The distressing and debilitating intestinal problems seen today have existed for centuries. The names given the various conditions with the symptoms of diarrhea, excess gas, loss of weight, excess mucus, cramping, blood loss, and severe constipation have changed throughout the years. The methods of diagnosis as well as those of treatment and management have also changed with time. But always, there has been a strong underlying belief that diet is an important factor to consider, not only in determining the causes of the disorders, but also in their treatment and cure.

The medical literature is rich with reports relating the favorable effects of dietary changes on the course of intestinal disease. As far back as 300 A.D., a Roman physician described in detail a diarrhea condition sounding like celiac disease and suggested that fasting, along with the use of the juice of the plantain, a member of the banana family, would cure the disease.[1] In 1745, Prince Charles, the Young Pretender to the throne of England, suffered from ulcerative colitis and was said to have cured himself by adopting a milk-free diet.[2]

During the early 1900's, numerous physicians brought further insight to our understanding of the effect of food on intestinal problems. Dr. Christian Herter, a physician and professor at Columbia University, noted that in every case where children were wasting away with diarrhea and debilitation, proteins were well tolerated, fats were handled moderately well but carbohydrates (sugars and starches) were badly tolerated. He stated that ingestion of some carbohydrates almost invariably caused a relapse or a return of diarrhea after a period of improvement.[3,4] About that time, Dr. Samuel Gee, another world-renowned children's specialist, saw clearly several important facts that continue to be missed by modern researchers. Dr. Gee said that if the patient with intestinal disease could be cured at all, it would have to be by means of diet.[5] He added that milk was the least suitable food during intestinal problems and that highly starchy food (rice, corn, potatoes, grains) were unfit. Dr. Gee stated, "We must never forget that what the patient takes beyond his power to digest does harm." Any food, and particularly carbohydrate, given to a person with intestinal problems should, therefore, be a food that requires little or no digestion so that the digestive process itself will not stand in the way of the absorption of the carbohydrates. Contrary to what some may think, undigested (and, therefore, unabsorbed) carbohydrates are not passing harmlessly through the small intestine and colon and out in the feces but, somehow and somewhere in the digestive tract, are causing problems.

There is much recent evidence to support the hypothesis that the course of several forms of intestinal problems can be favorably changed by manipulating the types of carbohydrates ingested. Cystic fibrosis patients have responded remarkably well to the removal of certain carbohydrates from their diets, especially refined sugar (sucrose) and the milk sugar, lactose, as well as starch.[6-9] Lactose has been implicated over and over again in ulcerative colitis, Crohn's disease, and other types of intestinal disorders referred to as "functional" diarrhea.[10-13] The removal of lactose from the diets of patients with these problems has resulted in remarkable improvement.[14-18]

Crohn's disease research has yielded some dramatic results relating to carbohydrates in the diet. In the 1980's two reports appeared in the medical literature. The first reported the results of Drs. Von Brandes and Lorenz-Meyer of Marburg, West Germany who brought about remissions in twenty patients with Crohn's disease by forbidding foods and beverages containing refined carbohydrates, mainly sucrose and starch.[19] In the second study involving twenty patients with Crohn's disease, dietary changes involving the elimination of specific foods, particularly cereals and dairy products, resulted in sustained remissions. The physicians conducting the research concluded that "dietary manipulation might be an effective long-term therapeutic strategy for Crohn's disease."[20] Dr. Claude Morin of Hospital Sainte-Justine, Quebec, reported his results in treating four children who were suffering from long-standing Crohn's disease. When Dr. Morin administered, via a stomach tube, a synthetic elemental diet containing the monosaccharide glucose (a single sugar) as the main carbohydrate source, the children showed remarkable gains in both height and weight as well as remission of their symptoms.[21] Unlike sucrose, lactose, and starch, *glucose requires no digestion* and is, therefore, more likely to be absorbed by the cells of the small intestine. This "predigested" sugar can easily pass through the intestinal absorptive cells, enter the bloodstream, and nourish the body. Glucose in the synthetic elemental diet as well as glucose found in fruits and honey is not beyond the power of those with disturbed digestive systems to absorb.

Dr. Jan Van Eys of the University of Texas Cancer Center reaffirmed this principle by stating:

> The gastrointestinal mucosa (surface) of children is especially prone to damage from diarrhea and, as a result, disaccharide intolerance. The development of disaccharide-deficient formulae and of elemental diets gave a means by which physicians could allow patients to recover without drastic measures.[22]

Dr. Van Eys did not elaborate on the conditions that lead to the inability to digest double sugars (disaccharides) nor did he state how diarrhea is related to the problem of disaccharide digestion. More recently, however, Dr. J. Ranier Poley of Eastern Virginia Medical School has shown a link between diarrhea and the inability to digest starch and disaccharide sugars.[23] By microscopically examining the

intestinal surface of patients with various forms of diarrhea,
Dr. Poley found that most patients have lost the ability to
digest disaccharides because of excessive mucus production
by intestinal cells. An abnormally thick layer of surface
mucus appears to be preventing contact between the
disaccharides and the digestive enzymes of the absorptive
cells. Sugars that need digestion cannot be processed and,
therefore, will not be absorbed to provide nourishment for
the individual. Dr. Poley has shown this phenomenon to
take place in those suffering with celiac disease (gluten-
sensitive enteropathy), soy-protein intolerance, intolerance
to cow's milk protein, intractable diarrhea of infancy, chronic
diarrhea in children, parasitic infections of the intestine
(Giardia), cystic fibrosis of the pancreas, and Crohn's
disease.[23] Reasons for the production of excessive mucus
will be discussed in greater detail in the next chapter dealing
with intestinal microbes.

Carbohydrates (sugars and starches) will be discussed
in Chapter 5 in order to understand how some are more likely
than others to escape digestion and, therefore, absorption.
It will become clear that when this occurs, they remain in
the intestinal tract and are utilized by the microbial world
of the intestine which depend on this available carbohydrate

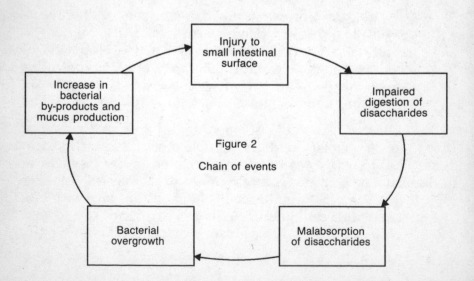

Figure 2

Chain of events

for the energy the microbes need to live and multiply.[24] Yeast and bacteria change the carbohydrates in ways that can injure the intestine which may respond to these microbial by-products by secreting excessive mucus. A chain of events (Figure 2) is then established.

At present, it is difficult to pinpoint the first step that triggers the cycle involving dietary carbohydrates and intestinal microbial growth. As far back as 1922, in a speech to the medical community entitled, "Faulty Food in Relation to Gastrointestinal Disorders," Dr. Robert McCarrison warned his colleagues that intestinal diseases were increasing. He asked them to remember that microbes, often blamed for intestinal disease, are dependent upon the conditions of life, especially nutrition, which "frequently prepare the soil of the body for the growth of these microorganisms."[25] It is reasonable to believe that undigested, unabsorbed carbohydrates remaining in the intestine can serve as "the soil of the body" which encourages the growth of microorganisms involved in intestinal disorders.

In various conditions, a poorly-functioning intestine can be easily overwhelmed by the ingestion of carbohydrates which require numerous digestive processes. The result is an environment that supports overgrowth of intestinal yeast and bacteria thus either initiating the chain of events or perpetuating it.

The purpose of the Specific Carbohydrate Diet is to deprive the microbial world of the intestine of the food it needs to overpopulate. By using a diet which contains predominantly "predigested" carbohydrates, the individual with an intestinal problem can be maximally nourished without over-stimulation of the intestinal microbial population.

Chapter 3

INTESTINAL MICROBES: THE UNSEEN WORLD

The two most hazardous things an astronaut takes into his capsule on extended flight are his brain and his intestinal flora.† (Bengson)[1]

A man is only what his microbes make him. (Kopeloff)[2]

It is generally accepted among physicians and researchers that during intestinal upsets and chronic intestinal disease, the normal, harmonious state of balance between intestinal microbes living in our gastrointestinal tract is lost. It is important, therefore, that we have some understanding of the inhabitants of our unseen world.

Before birth, the human intestine is free of microbes.[3,4] From the moment of birth, however, a massive invasion of the gastrointestinal tract takes place and it soon becomes populated with various types of microbes depending on the type of milk ingested as well as other environmental factors. Some of the microbial growth develops from contact with the mother's skin; some originates from the air. If the infant is breastfed, more than 99% of all microbes in the intestine are of one type.[3] As other foods are introduced, the baby develops a wide variety of bacteria.

† intestinal flora - the various bacterial and other microscopic forms of life in the intestinal contents.

Studies have revealed that eventually more than four hundred bacterial species live together in the human colon.[52] The stomach and most of the small intestine do not normally harbor more than a sparse population of microbial flora. However, the number of microbes normally increases at the lowest part of the small intestine, the ileum, because of its close proximity to the microbial-rich colon. [5

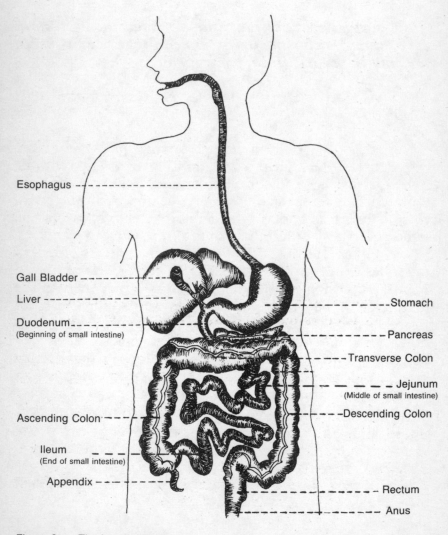

Figure 3   The intestinal tract

In the healthy intestinal tract, intestinal microbes appear to live in a state of balance; an overabundance of one type seems to be inhibited by the activities of other types. This competition between microbes prevents any one type from overwhelming the body with its waste products or toxins. Another important protective factor which works to maintain the sparse bacterial population of the stomach and upper small intestine is the high acidity of the stomach's hydrochloric acid in which microbes cannot usually survive. In addition, normal peristalsis (waves of involuntary muscular contractions) sweeps many microbes out of the intestine to be lost in the feces, thereby, decreasing their numbers.

However, bacterial overgrowth in the stomach and small intestine can and does occur for various reasons among which are:

(1) Interference with the high acidity of the stomach through the continual use of antacids;

(2) A decrease in the acidity of the stomach such as occurs in the aging process[6];

(3) Malnutrition or a diet of poor quality, and the resulting weakening of the body's immune system[7,8];

(4) Antibiotic therapy which can cause a wide range of microbial changes. A microbe commonly residing in the intestine without harmful effects may undergo a wide range of changes as a result of antibiotic therapy.[9]

Once the normal equilibrium of the colon is disturbed for any reason, its microbes can migrate into the small intestine and stomach hampering digestion, competing for nutrients, and overloading the intestinal tract with their waste products.[3] Quite early in bacterial overgrowth of the small intestine, the normal absorption of vitamin B_{12} is disturbed. There is considerable evidence that B_{12} is poorly absorbed when microbes multiplying within the small intestine prevent uptake by the ileum.[12,13]

There has been a long history indicating that bacteria and yeast are involved in intestinal disease. As far back as 1904, an examination of the stools of children who were suffering with what appeared to be celiac disease, revealed abnormally large numbers of fermentative (carbohydrate ''eaters'') and putrefactive (protein ''eaters'') bacteria which were, undoubtedly, contributing to the disease process. The physicians making this observation proposed that although the normal intestine controlled the growth of bacteria, in ''celiac-type'' cases some intestinal abnormality prevented the normal regulatory control.[14]

Early researchers working on ulcerative colitis believed this disorder to be caused by bacteria. From 1906 to 1924, numerous researchers isolated certain types of bacteria, injected either the bacteria or the bacterial toxins into laboratory animals, and claimed that the injections produced ulcerative colitis in the animals.[15-18] In 1932, when Dr. B.B. Crohn spoke about a ''new'' intestinal disorder which he called regional ileitis (now known as Crohn's disease), some physicians attending his lecture stated that this new disease entity might be due to microorganisms.[19]

From the 1920's until the present, the role of microbes and the products they produce continues to be investigated in an effort to find the cause of the various forms of inflammatory bowel disease.[20-26] Often there has been very convincing evidence that particular bacteria could initiate a certain type of intestinal disease but, eventually, the work has been dismissed because of insufficient proof. Some of the difficulties which these investigators experienced in trying to pinpoint the ''culprit'' microbes were undoubtedly due to the ever-changing conditions of the microbial world of the intestine, to variability in the strains of intestinal microbes, or to the lack of precise laboratory techniques of identification.

During these early years of investigation, Dr. Ilya Metchnikoff proposed that bacteria in the intestine were producing toxins which were then absorbed into the bloodstream. These toxins, Metchnikoff stated, were the cause of many human afflictions, and he named the process by which harmful microbes in the intestine cause disease, ''autointoxication''.[27] Unlike investigators who unsuccessfully attempted to find the precise microorganisms involved in the various types of intestinal disorders, Metchnikoff approached the problem quite differently. He maintained, as many others have done, that if the intestinal environment can be kept in a healthy state, harmful microbes will no longer be a threat.[30]

He advocated the widespread use of acidified (fermented) milk, similar to yoghurt, and proposed that the beneficial bacteria used in producing the fermented milk, and still remaining therein, would enter the intestinal tract and prevent other bacteria in the intestine from forming harmful toxins. While Metchnikoff's proposal has not been universally adopted, his ideas are acknowledged by outstanding gastroenterologists and researchers. In 1964, Dr. Donaldson stated in a lengthy article about the role of bacteria in intestinal disease, 'In certain respects the concept of autointoxication offered by Metchnikoff must now receive serious reconsideration'.[12]

Investigators continue to be fascinated by Metchnikoff's proposals and to study the potential benefits of acidified milk. Modern researchers are asking: Do the bacteria used to ferment the milk actually take up residence in the intestine and, if so, for how long? Which of the ''yoghurt-type'' bacteria used to acidify milk will counteract toxins produced by other intestinal microbes?[28] Is the bacteria used to acidify the milk or the acidified (fermented) milk itself the beneficial factor?[29]

In the 1980's an increasing number of reports have been published stating that intestinal bacterial toxins appear to be injuring intestinal cells and, as a result, causing a variety of diarrheal diseases. Some of the bacteria producing these toxins have not, in the past, been considered to be disease-causing types.[7] Although there is still insufficient evidence to link a specific microbe to each of the chronic intestinal disorders, it is generally agreed that intestinal microbes are not innocent bystanders.

A simple approach to minimizing the undesirable activities of intestinal microbes would seem to be through the use of antibiotics. This approach is often tried but, unfortunately, in most chronic intestinal disorders, it has limitations.[31-48]

We are faced, then, with intestinal disorders which involve microbial populations which have been altered in number, in kind, or both. The normal contractions (peristalsis) of the intestinal muscles are not able to remove them; they appear to be tenacious. Indeed, there is evidence that intestinal microbes will not cause disease unless they develop methods of adhering to the gut wall.[49,50] Antibiotic therapy is of limited usefulness while other drugs of the cortisone and sulfa families have side-effects if continued too long.

A sensible and harmless form of warfare on the aberrant population of intestinal microbes is to manipulate their energy (food) supply through diet. Most intestinal microbes require carbohydrates for energy,[51] and the Specific Carbohydrate Diet severely limits the availability of carbohydrates. By depriving intestinal microbes of their energy source, their numbers gradually decrease along with the products they produce.

Chapter 4

BREAKING THE VICIOUS CYCLE

Of all dietary components, carbohydrate has the major influence over intestinal microbes. Through a process of fermentation of available carbohydrates remaining in the intestinal tract, microbes obtain energy for continued maintenance and growth.[1]

The fermentation process by which intestinal microbes consume dietary carbohydrates is diagrammed below:

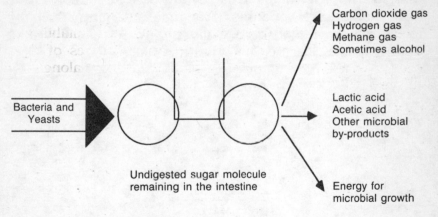

Carbon dioxide gas
Hydrogen gas
Methane gas
Sometimes alcohol

Bacteria and Yeasts

Lactic acid
Acetic acid
Other microbial
by-products

Undigested sugar molecule remaining in the intestine

Energy for microbial growth

Figure 4   Intestinal fermentation

Fermentation is encouraged when the diet contains carbohydrates which remain in the intestinal tract rather than being absorbed into the bloodstream.[2] Unabsorbed carbohydrates constitute the most important source of gas in the intestine. For example, the lactose contained in one ounce of milk, if undigested and unabsorbed, will produce about 50 ml of gas in the intestine of normal people. But under abnormal conditions when intestinal microbes have moved into the small intestine, the hydrogen gas production may be increased over one hundred-fold.

The presence of undigested and unabsorbed carbohydrates within the small intestine can encourage microbes from the colon to take up residence in the small intestine and to continue to multiply. This, in turn, may lead to the formation of products, in addition to gas, which injure the small intestine. Examples are lactic, acetic, and other acids (Fig. 4) which are short-chain organic acids resulting from the fermentative process. In addition to the damage to the intestine, there is a growing body of scientific evidence that lactic acid formed from fermentation in the intestine causes abnormal brain function and behavior,[3,4,5] which could account for the behavioral problems which often accompany intestinal disorders. This would also explain the dramatic improvements in behavior noted in Chapter 1: the formation of large amounts of lactic acid resulting from the fermentation of unabsorbed carbohydrates is prevented by following the Specific Carbohydrate Diet.

Figure 5   The vicious cycle

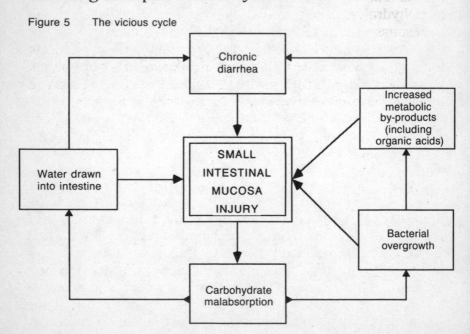

Once bacteria multiply within the small intestine, the chain of events diagrammed in Figure 5 develops into a vicious cycle characterized by an increase in the production of gas, acids and other products of fermentation which perpetuate the malabsorption problem and prolong the intestinal disorder.[6]

Bacterial growth in the small intestine appears to destroy the enzymes on the intestinal cell surface preventing carbohydrate digestion and absorption and making carbohydrates available for further fermentation.[7] It is at this point that production of excessive mucus may be triggered as a self-defense mechanism whereby the intestinal tract attempts to "lubricate" itself against the mechanical and chemical injury caused by the microbial toxins, acids, and the presence of incompletely digested and unabsorbed carbohydrates.

The Specific Carbohydrate Diet presents a method for breaking the cycle by maximally nourishing the individual and minimally nourishing the intestinal microbes. By this method, undesirable stresses on the intestine decrease. The diet is based on the principle that specifically selected carbohydrates, requiring minimal digestive processes (as will be discussed in Chapter 5) are absorbed and leave virtually none to be used for furthering microbial growth in the intestine. As the microbial population decreases due to lack of food, its harmful by-products also decrease, freeing the intestinal surface of injurious substances. No longer needing protection, the mucus-producing cells stop producing excessive mucus, and carbohydrate digestion is improved. Malabsorption is replaced by absorption. As the individual absorbs energy and nutrients, all the cells of the body are properly nourished, including the cells of the immune system, which then can assist in overcoming the microbial invasion. The practical Specific Carbohydrate Diet aims for the same goals as the clinical synthetic Elemental Diet: the reduction and change of bacterial growth and the maintenance of the optimum nutritional state of the patient.[9,10]

Chapter 5

CARBOHYDRATE DIGESTION

Digestion is the great secret of life. (Go and Summerskill)[1]

What the patient takes beyond his ability to digest does harm. (Gee)[2]

While the underlying causes of the various intestinal disorders cannot be stated with certainty, faulty digestion and malabsorption of dietary carbohydrates may be, in large part, responsible for these disorders. (Carbohydrate refers to starch and disaccharide sugar molecules; both require digestion before absorption.) As we have seen in previous chapters, this can lead to more serious malabsorption of all nutrients due to injury to the intestinal surface. The Specific Carbohydrate Diet most often corrects malabsorption allowing nutrients to enter the bloodstream and be made available to the cells of the body thereby strengthening the immune system's ability to fight. Further debilitation is prevented, weight can return to normal, and, ultimately, there is a return to health.

Malabsorption is the inability of the cells of the body to obtain nutrients from foods eaten. As a result, the caloric energy, vitamins, and minerals are lost as all parts of the body are deprived of the proper nourishment. There are many places in the gastrointestinal tract where problems could lead to malabsorption: (1) if food travels too rapidly through the intestinal tract (as happens most often when diarrhea is present), there is insufficient time for large food molecules such as starch, fat, and protein to be broken down by various enzymes and, consequently, their absorption into the bloodstream is seriously impaired; (2) if a poorly-functioning pancreas does not deliver sufficient digestive enzymes to the small intestine to break down large molecules of protein, fat, and starch, absorption of these nutrients will not take place.

However, a large number of research reports point to a later step in digestion as the site leading to malabsorption in many intestinal disorders.[4,5,8-14,16,18] This last step in the digestive process occurs at the microvilli of the cell membranes of the intestinal absorptive cell.

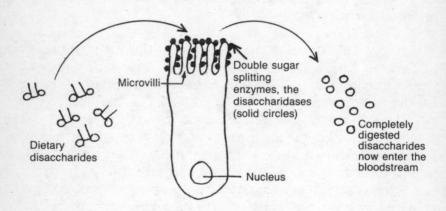

Figure 6   Tall, healthy, mature intestinal absorptive cell

The membranes of cells lining the intestinal tract serve as more than a passive barrier between the contents of the digestive tract and the bloodstream. When the digestive system is functioning normally, the membranes of these ''gatekeeper'' cells *actively* participate in the last step of digestion as well as aiding in the transport of nutrients into the bloodstream.

The last step in carbohydrate digestion takes place at the minute projections called microvilli (Fig. 6). Only those carbohydrates which have been properly processed by the enzymes embedded in the microvilli can cross over the

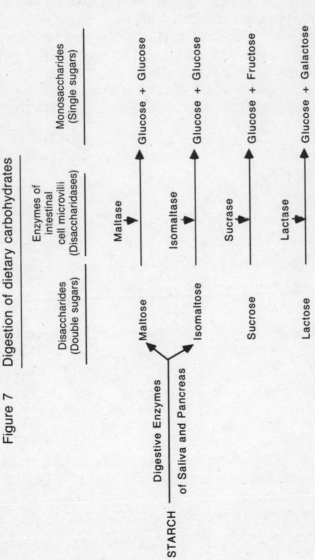

Figure 7　Digestion of dietary carbohydrates

barrier and enter the bloodstream.[3] This is where the milk sugar, lactose, and sucrose, are split apart (digested). This is also the site of the last step in the digestion of starch from such foods such as grains and potatoes. Figure 7 summarizes the steps involved in carbohydrate digestion in the gastrointestinal tract and lists the microvilli enzymes which carry out the last step of the digestive process.

The structure of the intestinal surface is dramatically altered during intestinal disease[4] and, as a result, digestive activity is seriously inhibited. This makes the last step in the digestion of these carbohydrates difficult, if not impossible[4-12,15] (Fig. 8)

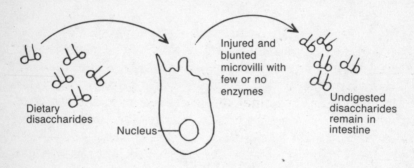

Figure 8   Flattened, injured, immature absorptive cell

The location of the sugar-splitting enzymes, the disaccharidases, in the membranes of the intestinal cells makes them very vulnerable to damage from many sources. A vitamin deficiency of folic acid [29], for example, and/or of B_{12}, can prevent proper development of the microvilli which carry the disaccharidases. An abnormally thick layer of mucus produced by the intestinal cells can prevent contact between the microvilli enzymes and the disaccharides lactose, sucrose, maltose and isomaltose.[4] In addition, irritating or toxic substances produced by yeast, bacteria, or parasities which have invaded the small intestinal tract can cause damage to the intestinal cell membranes, destroying their enzymes.[13]

Conditions involving the small intestine that are frequently associated with deficiencies of lactase and other disaccharidases are celiac disease, malnutrition, tropical sprue, cholera, gastroenteritis, infant diarrhea from any cause, pellagra, irritable colon, post-gastrectomy (removal of part of stomach),[14] soy protein intolerance, intolerance to cow's milk protein, intractable diarrhea of infancy, parasitic infections of the intestine, cystic fibrosis, and Crohn's disease.[4,5,8-14,16,18] In addition, lactase deficiency in ulcerative colitis is well documented as was noted in Chapter 2.

The first enzyme to suffer damage is usually lactase, but often there is a combination of enzyme loss involving sucrase, isomaltase, and, less often, maltase.[14] The enzyme, lactase, is depressed earlier than the other disaccharide-splitting enzymes in intestinal disturbances such as celiac disease (and other conditions where diarrhea is present) and is the last of the microvilli enzymes to return to normal after intestinal disease has subsided. In fact, lactase may be permanently depressed after severe malnutrition and tropical diarrhea (sprue) and a deficiency of lactase may be the sole legacy of some previous disorders.[14]

It is difficult to prove the absence of disaccharidase activity by present medical techniques. A biopsy sample of the small intestine during intestinal disease may show that enzyme activity of disaccharidases is normal. However, upon feeding lactose, sucrose, and starch, cramping, diarrhea, and vomiting will follow. This apparent contradiction could be due to a lack of contact between the enzymes and sugars caused by the mucus barrier referred to in Chapters 2 and 3.

When a biopsy sample *does* indicate that there is a deficiency of disaccharidase enzyme activity, the reason could be a primary genetic problem or a secondary problem caused by a direct injury to the intestinal cell surface with loss of the microvilli and a flattening of the cell itself. Among those factors which lead to injuries of the intestinal surface are malnutrition and irritation caused by substances produced by microbial growth.[15,16]

The sugars, then, remain undigested in the small intestine.[4,17] Their presence in the lumen (interior space) of the intestine causes a reversal of the normal nutritional process. Instead of nutrients flowing from the intestinal space into the bloodstream, water is drawn into the intestinal lumen (Fig. 5). The water, carrying nutrients, is lost in abnormal intestinal function (diarrhea) and the cells of the body are deprived of energy, minerals, and vitamins. Most seriously, the sugars remaining in the intestinal lumen provide energy for further fermentation and growth of intestinal microbes.

The increasing levels of irritating substances given off by the growing microbial population cause intestinal cells to defend themselves. Mucus-producing cells (goblet cells) which are normally present in the intestine secrete their product to cover and protect the naked free surface of the intestinal absorptive cells. The small intestine responds to a disruption of the normal balance by producing more goblet cells which increases the secretion of intestinal mucus. As the integrity of the small intestine is further threatened by the microbial invasion and by the products it produces, a thick mucus barrier forms for self defense. The enzymes embedded within the absorptive cell membranes cannot do the job for which they are designed: to make contact with and split certain sugars in the diet.[4]

If the goblet cells become exhausted (and there is a limit to their valiant efforts to defend the absorptive lining against irritation), the "naked" intestinal surface is subject to further ravaging. It is very possible that, at this stage, ulceration of the intestinal surface, as seen in ulcerative colitis, can occur. This might also explain how certain proteins such as gluten can inappropriately enter the interior of the absorptive cells and destroy them.

Sometimes, but not often, even the absorption of single sugars is disturbed because of severe injury to the absorptive cells, but this extreme condition is usually diagnosed by routine hospital tests.[18] Sometimes, the invasion of microbes into the small intestine is so pervasive that yeast, for example, will be found in the esophagus.[19]

When it is suspected that yeast invasion is widespread (the oral infection, thrush, would be an indicator) it is wise to cut back on honey ingestion at the beginning of the dietary regimen (amount of honey in recipes should be decreased by at least 75%). The amount of honey may be increased as the condition improves.

The indigestibility of starch by even healthy people is only recently receiving attention (see descriptions of starches following). Some starchy foods which were assumed to be digested completely are, in fact, incompletely digested by most people.[20,21] In those people with intestinal disorders, the digestibility of starch is even further affected. Because the breakdown of starch eventually results in the formation of the disaccharides, maltose and isomaltose, most starches must be avoided unless they are specified as permissible in Chapter 8.

Some foods in the Specific Carbohydrate Diet contain starches which have been shown to be tolerated. These are the starches of the legume family: dried beans, lentils and split peas (no chick peas, soybeans or bean sprouts). The legumes which are permitted must, however, be soaked for at least 10-12 hours prior to cooking and the water discarded since they contain other sugars which are indigestible but which can be removed by soaking.[22] The legumes may be introduced in small amounts at about the third month of the diet. The starches in all grains, corn, and potatoes must be strictly avoided. Corn syrup is also excluded since it contains a mixture of ''short-chain'' starches.[23,24]

Carbohydrates Found in Foods

1. Single Sugars (monosaccharides)

These sugars require no further splitting in order to be transported from the intestine into the bloodstream. They are glucose, fructose, and galactose. Glucose and fructose are found in honey, fruits, and some vegetables. Galactose is found in lactose-hydrolyzed milk (LHM) and in yoghurt.

2. Double Sugars (disaccharides)

These sugars require splitting by intestinal cell enzymes. There are four main disaccharides: lactose, sucrose, maltose, and isomaltose.

Lactose is found in fluid milk, dried milk powder, commercial yoghurt, homemade yoghurt which has not been fermented for twenty-four hours, processed cheeses, cottage cheese, cream cheese, ice cream, some sour creams, whey (70% lactose by weight), and many products which have added milk solids or whey. Many drugs and vitamin and mineral supplements have added lactose.

Sucrose is table sugar and is found in processed foods such as gelatin desserts, ketchup, cereals, many canned foods and some frozen preparations (see Appendix). There is a small amount of sucrose (about 1%-3%) in some pasteurized honey but it has been shown to be tolerated by those on the Specific Carbohydrate Diet. Unpasteurized honey contains virtually no sucrose since an enzyme in the honey splits whatever sucrose may be present. Some fruits and nuts contain small amounts of sucrose but they may be used and have been included in Chapter 8. As fruits ripen, some of the sucrose they may contain is split by enzymes within the fruit.

Maltose and Isomaltose are found in sources such as corn syrup, malted milk, and candies. However, most of the maltose and isomaltose which is presented to the intestinal cells for digestion comes from dietary starches. Starches are long chains of glucose molecules (Fig. 9) which are digested, in part, by enzymes from the pancreas and saliva and are left as the disaccharides, maltose and isomaltose, to be split by microvilli enzymes of intestinal cells.

3. Starch (polysaccharides) can be of two types called amylose and amylopectin. Most vegetables contain both types in various proportions. For example, some kinds of rice contain small amounts of amylopectin starch and large

amounts of amylose starch. Other types of rice contain only amylopectin starch.[25] Like rice, some genetic strains of corn contain a very highly branched amylopectin type of starch. Sweet potatoes or yams also contain only amylopectin starch. It appears that genetic breeding which attempts to change the protein content of certain crops also affects the types of starch formed by the plant.[25] The varying proportions of different kinds of starch might affect the ability of the intestine to completely digest them. Or, as will be discussed in Chapter 6, the proteins of certain plants may prevent the starch from being completely split.[27] (It is interesting to note that one group of researchers have found that some intestinal bacteria are made more virulent by the presence of undigested cornstarch in the intestine.[26])

Vegetables that contain more amylose than amylopectin starch are simpler to digest, because the glucose units which make up all starch molecules are arranged in a linear fashion in amylose starch and are readily exposed to digestive enzymes from saliva and the pancreas (Fig. 9). The links holding the glucose units in these linear arrays

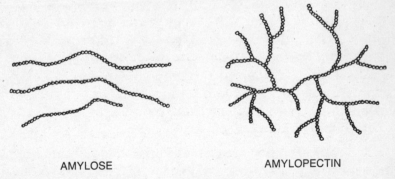

AMYLOSE   AMYLOPECTIN

Each small circle in the above diagrams represents a glucose molecule.

Figure 9   Starches

are split until the chains are reduced to only two chemically linked glucose molecules called maltose. By comparison, amylopectin molecules contain glucose units which form branches (Figs. 9 and 10). When the amylopectin molecules have been partially digested by pancreatic enzymes, the fragments remaining for the last step in digestion by microvilli enzymes are both maltose and isomaltose.

Recently, Dr. Gunja-Smith and associates proposed that the amylopectin starch molecule is even more highly branched than was thought originally.[28]

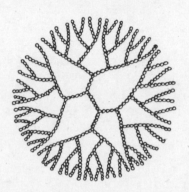

Figure 10   Revised diagram of amylopectin starch

According to Dr. Gunja-Smith's diagram, the interior branches appear less exposed than the exterior branches. It is, therefore, possible that pancreatic digestive enzymes cannot reach the interior links and that parts of the amylopectin starch molecules escape digestion, remain in the intestine, and increase microbial fermentation.

At present, very limited information is available as to the amounts of amylopectin and amylose starch present in the many kinds of grains and other starchy foods.

Fiber. Fruits, vegetables, nuts, and grains contain various components, termed fiber, which are indigestible by the enzymes of the digestive tract. Fiber from fruits, nuts, vegetables, including dried legumes, is allowed on the Specific Carbohydrate Diet but all other fiber from grains, including bran, is not permitted.

Chapter 6

BEYOND GLUTEN

Grains, including wheat, rye, oats, corn, barley, rice, and buckwheat have been viewed with suspicion in the management of intestinal disorders, especially in the treatment of celiac disease. Before the 1950's, it was felt that their adverse effect on intestinal cells was due to the starchy components of the grains. In 1950, however, a Dutch researcher, W. K. Dicke, proposed that the protein constituent of wheat, the gluten, produced permanent injury to the intestinal cells of those people suffering from celiac disease.[1]

Gluten is the predominant protein in wheat and rye and like all proteins, it is composed of hundreds of building blocks called amino acids which are linked together to form the protein molecule. In most people, the gluten molecule is broken down by digestive enzymes in the small intestine and the simple amino acids of which gluten is composed are absorbed by the intestinal absorptive cells to provide nutrition for the rest of the body.[2,3] It is believed that this is not the case in celiac disease and that the gluten remains undigested.

Before the 1950's, a celiac patient was usually diagnosed according to the clinical symptoms the patient exhibited. In children, for example, their growth and weight would be below normal, they would display a distended abdomen although the rest of their bodies were quite thin, and they would suffer with frequent episodes of diarrhea alternating with periods of normal stools and constipation. The stools would have a pale and greasy appearance with a foul odor. Based on these signs and additional laboratory tests, the diagnosis of celiac disease would be made. The patient would be placed on protein milk (with no lactose), with the elimination of certain starchy foods as well as sucrose- and lactose-containing foods and within a short time, all symptoms would disappear for good.[4]

Dr. Dicke's thesis, combined with a new diagnostic tool, the intestinal biopsy instrument, developed into a new approach to identifying celiac disease. In spite of the presenting symptoms, the patient would not be diagnosed as a celiac until certain other criteria were met. A series of intestinal biopsies would be done: one tissue sample would be taken from the small intestine before gluten was removed from the diet; a second sample would be taken after the patient had been on a gluten-free diet, a third biopsy sample would be taken after the patient was challenged with gluten. The biopsy samples would have to reflect the changes in the diet: When viewed under the microscope, the intestinal cells would have to appear flattened or blunted while the person ingested gluten; after gluten withdrawal, the cells would have to change into tall, efficient absorptive cells; and, upon the reintroduction of gluten, the cells would have to revert to the flattened type. If a patient fulfilled this established criteria, his condition would then be given the name, ''gluten-induced enteropathy celiac disease.'' Thus, only a small number of persons exhibiting the clinical symptoms of malabsorption including diarrhea, bloated belly, and failure to thrive could now be classified as true celiacs. The remainder, a large group with the same clinical symptoms as the others, would be said to be suffering from such conditions as idiopathic (from unknown causes) diarrhea, tropical sprue (diarrhea of the tropics), non-tropical sprue, steatorrhea (fat in the stool), failure-to-thrive syndrome, or malabsorption. Therefore, if a physician applied the strict definition for diagnosing celiac disease, the number of ''true'' celiacs would remain very small with a large group of patients with different diagnoses.[5]

Many members of the medical community welcomed the new diagnositic approach for it appeared that the real culprit in grains had been identified and that the biopsy samples were proof of the sought-after "cause-and-effect" phenomenon. Furthermore, only one food component, gluten, would have to be eliminated, simplifying the difficult problem of keeping people on a more restricted diet.

Unfortunately, things were not so simple. It soon became apparent that grains which contained proteins other than gluten were having deleterious effects on the intestinal cells. At the same time, corn, containing large amounts of gluten, appeared to be tolerated. Some patients suffered relapses and exhibited damaged intestinal cells (microscopically) upon eating soy products.[6,7] Oats and barley were found to contain gluten-like proteins which offended many celiac sufferers.[8] British clinics, therefore, have customarily eliminated wheat, rye, barley, and oats and have allowed rice and corn. Additional reports, however, have implicated rice as well as the other grains as being harmful to intestinal cells.[9,10]

Despite extensive research by many investigators, there is as yet no certainty about the precise nature of the gluten which is causing injury to the intestinal cells. During the 1970's, as newer techniques permitted researchers to further subdivide the large gluten molecule into smaller fractions, it was found that the alpha-gliadin fraction possessed toxic properties which appeared to injure intestinal cells of the true celiacs.[5] But there still remain unanswered questions about this smaller alpha-gliadin protein fraction: (1) Is there a genetic lack of the digestive enzymes which would normally split these gliadin molecules into their single amino acids thereby preventing their harmful effects? (2) Is there a weakness in the membranes of the intestinal cells which permits the intact, undigested gliadin molecules to penetrate the intestinal cells and, once inside, "poison" the cells? (3) Do the gliadin molecules bind to the surface of the intestinal cells and, thereby, immobilize the cells and destroy them? The most popular theory is that

the gliadin fraction, by penetrating the intestinal cell
membrane, reaches the underlying layer of white blood cells
and causes an immune response. The products of the
immune response, including antibodies, injure the intestinal
cells and cause them to change their shape and to function
abnormally.[5] More recent findings have implicated a
carbohydrate molecule attached to the gliadin molecule as
the toxic compound. When the carbohydrate is removed,
the gliadin molecule is no longer injurious to the intestinal
cells.[11,12]

Very recent research has cast more light on the
gluten-celiac hypothesis and highlights the interaction
between the starch and protein components of flour milled
from grains. Almost all normal people fail to absorb a large
amount of the starch of wheat flour.[29] This incomplete
absorption of starch results in an increase in intestinal
fermentation and the production of intestinal gas. In an effort
to discover why wheat starch is not completely digested by
many people, investigations were conducted relating to the
physical structure of wheat flour. It was found that wheat
flour is composed of granules containing a starch core
surrounded by a network of gluten protein. This protein-
starch complex can be separated by a manufacturing process
whereby most of the gluten is removed. The remaining flour
is sold as low-gluten flour and when it is substituted for
regular wheat flour, there is improvement in starch digestion
and absorption. Surprisingly, when the low gluten flour is
baked into bread **together with the separated gluten**,
starch malabsorption does not occur in spite of the fact that
the same amount of gluten is present in the baked product
as was present in the whole grain before gluten extraction.
Since absorption of the wheat starch is complete, there is
no resulting fermentation and intestinal gas. This indicates
that it is not the gluten alone which results in intestinal
symptoms.[29]

The investigators feel that it is the interaction
between the starch and the gluten which results in the
incomplete digestion and incomplete absorption of starch

and which causes intestinal gas, abdominal discomfort, and diarrhea. They speculate that the gluten extraction process alters or exposes the starch core thereby making the starch more vulnerable to pancreatic digestive enzymes.[13,29] This intriguing interaction between the starch and protein of grains will, undoubtedly, be the basis for much future research and may be shown to have some bearing on those with celiac disease.

Often patients show remarkable clinical improvement in their general well-being after following a gluten-free diet. However, biopsy samples, as viewed under the microscope, show intestinal cells that are still markedly abnormal.[14] It is, therefore, becoming increasingly clear that certain patients who have qualified as "true celiacs" and who have had gluten removed from their diets do not always show improvement on the cellular level. To further confound diagnosis, some patients who start eating gluten suffer no ill effects at one time but become extremely ill at other times. Thus, not only do different celiac patients vary in their response to gluten-free diets but the same patient may vary from time to time.[16]

The reaction to these inconsistencies has been that diagnosis must become more precise and, therefore, additional intestinal biopsies must be taken to confirm or deny that gluten is the underlying problem.[15]

But even the underlying basis for diagnosing "true celiacs" according to the appearance of the intestinal biopsy tissue under the microscope has been seriously questioned. The flattened or blunted intestinal surface has been reported in innumerable disease states: infectious hepatitis, ulcerative colitis, parasitic infections of the intestine, including various types of worms and one-celled parasites, kwashiorkor,[17] and in conditions such as soy protein intolerance, intolerance to cow's milk protein, intractable diarrhea of infancy, Crohn's disease,[18] and even after strict reducing diets by obese people.[17] Bacterial overgrowth of the small intestine has also resulted in patchy broadening and flattening of the small intestinal surface.[19] Just about all conditions associated with diarrhea seem to result in the same appearance of the small intestine as is seen in the so-called ''true celiac''. It seems, then, that the flattening of the intestinal cells is a secondary occurrence resulting from some other primary cause and is, in fact, seen during many conditions, especially when diarrhea is present.[20,21]

The most disquieting development in the gluten-celiac picture is the fact that celiacs, whether or not they respond favorably or unfavorably to gluten withdrawal, exhibit other serious intestinal problems which a gluten-free diet does not appear to be effective in preventing.[14,22] It seems, therefore, that something other than the protein, gluten, is involved in the underlying cause of the disorder.

Some investigators have always maintained that an inability to digest disaccharides induces the sensitivity to gluten.[23] But even were the disaccharides not the underlying cause of gluten intolerance, these double sugars should not be included in the diet of celiacs.[23] The flattened intestinal absorptive cells have lost their ability to perform the last step in digestion which is to split disaccharides.[18,24] Many researchers have confirmed the fact that in celiac patients, ability to digest disaccharides, especially lactose, is severely limited.[18,25-27] To include disaccharides and certain starches in the diet of those exhibiting a flattened intestinal surface is to demand the impossible of these digestive and absorptive cells and to add to the existing problems.[28]

The Specific Carbohydrate Diet has been shown to completely cure most cases of celiac disease if followed for at least one year.[4] It is truly a gluten-free diet, eliminating all grains which contain gluten or gluten-like proteins while also recognizing the limitations of the injured intestinal surface.

Chapter 7

INTRODUCING THE DIET

One basic principle of the diet must be firmly established and persistently repeated: no food should be ingested that contains carbohydrates other than those found in fruits, honey, properly-prepared yoghurt, and those vegetables and nuts listed. While this principle may be clearly understood, it is sometimes difficult in practice to recognize the existence of carbohydrates in various foods. Small quantities of carbohydrates other than those designated often creep into the diet unless the strictest attention is paid to every item of food.[1] Reading labels, although a good policy, is inadequate for those on the Specific Carbohydrate Diet since one ingredient sometimes has numerous names and may not be easily recognized as a forbidden carbohydrate. Many cans, jars, bottles, and packages do not list all ingredients because of different labeling laws in different parts of the country. *It is recommended that nothing be eaten other than those foods listed in Chapter 8.*

Because fruits and raw vegetables have qualities which tend to make them laxative, they must be used with care when diarrhea is still active. Although all fruits, all raw vegetables, and as much honey as desired may be used when the diarrhea has cleared, it is best to eliminate them until that time. When fruits are introduced, after a week or two, they should be ripe, peeled, and cooked. Raw fruits should not be introduced until diarrhea is under control. Raw vegetables such as salad greens, carrots and celery sticks, cucumbers, and onions also should not be introduced until diarrhea is under control.

Ripe, mashed banana is one of the uncooked fruits which may be tried first. Start cautiously with about one-quarter banana the first day. Only fully ripe bananas with no trace of green at the tips, the skin well-speckled with brown, and the edible portion soft enough to mash easily should be used. Most of the carbohydrate in the unripe banana is in the form of starch which is converted, in the process of ripening, to monosaccharide sugars which are easily absorbable by those with malabsorption problems.

Most canned fruits are forbidden because of the added sugar. If cooked fruits are desired, they may be prepared at home with saccharin or honey. Artificial sweeteners other than saccharin should be avoided. It is interesting to note that saccharin has been vindicated as far as bladder cancer is concerned.[2]

Low calorie diet foods often contain sorbitol or xylitol as sweeteners. Occasionally low calorie diet chewing gum or candy containing these sweeteners may be used. However, excessive use of these products can cause diarrhea and bloating.[5]

The Specific Carbohydrate Diet includes dairy products although fluid milk and some commercial products are eliminated. A list of the many cheeses which are allowed can be found in the Appendix along with those cheeses which are not permitted. Homemade yoghurt, prepared according to instructions found in the recipe section, is permitted. It is very important that the yoghurt instructions be followed precisely so that virtually none of its lactose remains. This is particularly true for the length of fermentation; *a minimum of 24 hours is required.* Another dairy product which should be included is *dry curd* cottage cheese. Every effort should be made to obtain this high-protein, sugar-free cheese for which the dairy man in your local market should help you find a source. It is not acceptable if it has any form of added milk or cream. Dry curd cottage cheese is a very important part of the diet since it may be "creamed" with homemade yoghurt and substituted for regular cottage cheese, it may be used as a base for pancakes and cheese cake, and it may be used for short periods as an infant formula (see Gourmet Section).

WARNING: Some dairies are calling a type of cottage cheese (with added milk products) ''uncreamed'' since there is very little fat (cream) in the milk which has been added. This type of cottage cheese is **not** permitted. It is quite moist, contains a considerable amount of lactose, and should immediately be recognized as not being a **dry** curd.

It is not advisable to use lactose-hydrolyzed milk (LHM) either prepared in the home or as a commercially available product at the beginning of the dietary regimen. Although lactose-hydrolyzed milk decreases fermentation in the intestine, its effect on the liver of those with chronic intestinal disorders has yet to be investigated. Additional research should be conducted to determine the speed with which the sugars of LHM milk reach the liver. Only then will it be known if the blood galactose (one of the sugars in LHM) stays within normal levels or rises too high.[3] Once the individual makes considerable progress and is on the road to recovery, small amounts of LHM may be used in tea, coffee and in cooking.

When brisk diarrhea is no longer present, egg may be added to the diet. When bowel movements are formed and occur no more than two or three times daily, cooked vegetables may be added to the diet cautiously, one at a time, with a sufficient period between each new introduction to determine its effect. In some instances diarrhea recurs when vegetables or fruits are given, in which case their use must be postponed. In general, squash, tomato, string beans, and carrots, all in cooked form, are well tolerated. Canned vegetables are not permitted because many have added sugar or starch which the labels often do not indicate. Potatoes and yams are not permitted.

Fats in association with meats, in butter, cheese, and in homemade yoghurt are well tolerated. It is usually not necessary to use skim or 2% milk unless one is eliminating fats in order to lose weight or because of some other health problem.

The Specific Carbohydrate Diet is highly nutritious and, depending on the choice of foods, is well-balanced. Every effort should be made to "round-out" the diet by eating sensibly and not, for example, consuming large quantities of meat or more than four muffins each day *to the exclusion of other foods*.

The diet should be discussed with your physician. Medication should continue as the physician has instructed. As progress is made, the physician, undoubtedly, will reduce medication gradually. WARNING: There are very specific procedures by which certain medications are reduced and it can be dangerous to discontinue their use improperly. Always seek medical advice in reducing medication.

As is advisable for all people, a daily diet should consist of a variety of foods: vegetables, fruits, cheeses, nuts, and some animal products. However, if one desires a diet without animal products, it is possible to eliminate them. The many essential nutrients which one gives up when on a strict vegetarian diet must be considered. It is beyond the scope of this book to include lists of foods which are rich in iron and B_{12}, two nutrients which are difficult to get in a strict vegetarian diet, and it is the responsibility of those who choose vegetarianism to see that other foods replace the nutrients given up when one eliminates animal products. Since soy products, including tofu, are not permitted on this diet, it will be very difficult, but possible, for a strict vegetarian to obtain sufficient nutrients and calories.

Most people with chronic intestinal disorders also suffer from malabsorption and, consequently, are malnourished. It is advisable that they add a vitamin supplement that specifically states that it is free of sugar, starch, and yeast (see Appendix). It may be necessary to write to the company manufacturing the vitamin to be sure of the ingredients. Any supplement such as bee pollen or herbs must be carefully checked since many companies have used whey (70% lactose), sugars, or starches as fillers and binding substances.

In the winter, in northern climates, vitamin D should be taken in combination with vitamin A as cod-liver or halibut-oil (400 I.U. Vitamin D and 5000 I.U. Vitamin A). For people who cannot tolerate the oils, even in capsule form, there are excellent substitutes in the form of water-soluble Vitamins A and D.

The malabsorption of Vitamin B_{12} is very often a part of chronic intestinal disorders and a special effort should be made, often by injections by the physician, to bring B_{12} levels up to **high normal**. There is some evidence that low levels, although they fall within the "normal" range, are not ideal for optimal health.

The B-Complex vitamins: B_1, B_2, Niacinamide, B_6, Pantothenic Acid, Folic Acid, Biotin, and B_{12} may be taken as a supplement (all in one tablet). Too much Folic Acid should be avoided; the amount taken should range from about 0.1-0.8 mg. Folic Acid and B_{12} work in unison in the cells of the body and it is important not to take more than 0.4 mg Folic Acid unless one is positive that B_{12} levels are in the high normal range; only then may one take up to 0.8 mg.

Any woman with an intestinal disorder who is on the contraceptive pill must very seriously consider vitamin supplementation, especially of the B-Complex family of vitamins, some of which are depleted by birth control medication.

Since Vitamin C is readily destroyed as a result of cooking and exposure to air, it is advisable that at least 100 mg be taken daily. If larger amounts of Vitamin C are currently being taken, one may continue provided that there is no starch or sugar in the Vitamin C preparation and that one is certain that the higher doses are not contributing to diarrhea.

It is the belief of the author that very large doses of added vitamins are unnecessary; the diet is highly nutritious and vitamin supplements are used in moderation to help in the recovery. Added minerals may be in order but it is very difficult to obtain satisfactory mineral supplements.

While cells of the body require approximately twenty different minerals, most mineral supplements contain only about eight. Since minerals compete with each other for absorption by the intestinal cells, it is possible that by taking a few, rather than all twenty, one could upset the delicate balance which, ideally, would be obtained from a nutritious diet. However, since many people with intestinal disorders are malnourished, it would be wise to check with your physician concerning the levels of the important minerals such as calcium, iron, iodine, and potassium. If mineral levels are low, they may be taken for a short time until malabsorption is corrected. Minerals, unlike vitamins, are not destroyed by air or temperature but can be lost in cooking water. Once malabsorption is corrected, the superb nutrition of the Specific Carbohydrate Diet should supply adequate minerals.

NOTE: Maintaining proper calcium levels is extremely important, especially in babies and growing children. The infant formula in the Gourmet Section provides calcium but not as much as is found in fluid milk or yoghurt. Therefore, if the infant formula is used for more than two weeks, blood calcium levels should be checked periodically by a physician who may suggest calcium supplementation.

It is impossible to specify the exact amount of vitamin supplementation necessary for each individual. These formulations are offered as reasonable amounts. Please check with your doctor.

For children:

Vitamin A	5000 IU+	Vitamin B_1	1.5-5 mg
Vitamin D	400 IU	Vitamin B_2	1.5-5 mg
(not when getting summer sun)		Niacinamide	10-20 mg
Vitamin E	10-30 IU	Pantothenic Acid	2-5 mg
		Vitamin B_6	2-5 mg
Vitamin C	50 mg++	Biotin	30-100 ug+++
		Folic Acid	0.1-0.3 mg
		Vitamin B_{12}	0.6-3.0 ug

For adults:

Vitamin A	5000 IU	Vitamin B$_1$	10-15 mg
Vitamin D	400 IU	Vitamin B$_2$	10-15 mg
(not when getting summer sun)		Niacinamide	25-50 mg
Vitamin E	100 IU	Pantothenic Acid	10-15 mg
		Vitamin B$_6$	10-15 mg
Vitamin C	100-500 mg	Biotin	100-200 ug
		Folic Acid	0.1-0.5 mg
		Vitamin B$_{12}$	100-200 ug

+ International Units
++ milligrams
+++ micrograms

The listed values are approximations. It is sometimes difficult to get all members of the B-Complex family in one tablet. However, never purchase a B-Complex vitamin with only B$_1$, B$_2$, and Niacin. The minimal members of the B-Complex family which should be included are B$_1$, B$_2$, Niacin, Pantothenic Acid and B$_6$. It is wise to purchase the fat soluble vitamins (A, D, E) separately from other vitamins. Unless they are in separate containers, there is a tendency to continue taking Vitamin D in the summer which should not be done unless the individual is housebound or gets very little exposure to the sun.

In prescribing this diet it is almost more important to stress what is not eaten than what is eaten. **Any cereal grain is strictly and absolutely forbidden,** including corn, oats, wheat, rye, rice, millet, buckwheat, or triticale in any form, whether as bread, cake, toast, zweiback, crackers, cookies, cereals, flour, or pasta (spaghetti, macaroni, or pizza). New grain substitutes are being placed on the market frequently. Some such as amaranth, quinoa, and cottonseed contain carbohydrates of unknown analysis and are not recommended while on this diet. Cereal bran, in any form, is strictly forbidden because its indigestible fiber provides an overload of carbohydrates which are fermented by intestinal bacteria. In addition, most forms of cereal bran contain large amounts of starch.[4] White table sugar or brown sugar is forbidden as a sweetener or in forms such as candy, pastries, or breads.

The strictness of this diet cannot be overemphasized nor should the difficulty of adhering to it be minimized. Faithful observance requires intelligence and vigilance on the part of those taking care of the individual or on the part of the person who cooks for himself or herself. It is surprising how many times a child will manage, despite the best supervision, to get hold of forbidden food. It is equally surprising how many parents will decide, despite all warnings, that ''just a taste'' of ice cream, cookie, or candy will do no harm. Such infringements will seriously delay recovery and it is unwise to undertake this regimen unless you are willing to follow it with **fanatical adherence**.

Many people have approached the dietary program by planning to give it a one month trial. If followed carefully for only one month, there should be changes for the better. These improvements provide the encouragement and support needed to commit oneself for the necessary longer period. It is recommended that a chart be kept for this first month. Hang it in a convenient location, preferably the kitchen. Across the top of the sheet, list those symptoms which describe the condition such as gas, diarrhea, or nightmares. Down the side of the sheet, number each line for the days of the month. At the end of each day, fill in the chart. For example, ''four +'s'' could be used to describe a lot of gas for that day. If there is a little less the following day, ''three +'s'' could be filled in. At the end of the month, progress can be evaluated. At this point, a personal commitment can be made to continue for a year or more, depending upon the speed of recovery.

If you see no improvement after a one month trial, the diet will probably not work for you. It is your decision at this point to return to your old pattern of eating or to continue eating according to the outlined diet. Your decision, of course, will depend upon your overall state of well being.

At the beginning of the program, when symptoms such as diarrhea and cramping are severe, the following basic diet should be followed for about five days. In other cases, one or two days on this basic diet is sufficient. The amounts of the specified foods to be eaten depend upon the appetite of the individual; there is no restriction as to quantities eaten.

Breakfast: Dry cottage cheese (moistened with homemade yoghurt).
Eggs (boiled, poached, or scrambled).
Apple cider or grape juice (½ juice, ½ water). (See Appendix re juices).
Homemade gelatin made with juice, unflavored gelatin, sweetener.

Lunch: Homemade chicken soup including broth, chicken, puréed carrots (see page 62).
Broiled beef patty or broiled fish.
Cheese cake (see page 92) without lemon rind and baked to custard consistency.
Homemade gelatin.

Dinner: Variations of above

If a food specified in the diet is known to cause an anaphylactic reaction (severe allergic reaction) eliminate it permanently from the diet. If, in the past, an allowable food did not agree with you, eliminate it for a short time (about one week) and try it again in small amounts. If, after a week of eliminating it, a food continues to cause problems, do not include it in the diet.

If you find it impossible to obtain the dry curd cottage cheese, substitute the cream cheese recipe (drained homemade yoghurt) listed in the Gourmet Section.

When diarrhea and cramping subside, cooked fruit, banana, and additional vegetables may be tried. If they seem to cause additional gas or diarrhea when they are added to the diet, delay their use until later. As the individual begins to feel better, the rest of the diet may be introduced. Do not use vegetables in the cabbage family until diarrhea has substantially subsided. Dried legumes may be added cautiously after being on the diet for about three months.

Most cases begin to improve within three weeks after the dietary regimen has been started and improvement usually continues. At about the second or third month, there is sometimes a relapse even when the diet has been carefully followed. This can occur if the person develops a respiratory infection or for no obvious reason. Do not allow this to discourage you! Once the individual gets over this, improvement is usually steady with minor setbacks occurring occasionally during the first year.

Many cases of celiac disease, spastic colon, and diverticulitis appear to be cured by the end of a year. Other disorders such as Crohn's disease and ulcerative colitis take much longer with the minimum time of two years on the diet. A rule of thumb is to stay on the diet for at least one year after the last symptom has disappeared.

At that time, introduce one forbidden food at a time. It is advisable to add only one food per week, starting with very small amounts and increasing the amount as the week progresses. The next week, another food may be added. If these foods appear to be well tolerated, one may decide to return to a regular diet. If symptoms recur upon the introduction of a forbidden food, it is best to remain on the Specific Carbohydrate Diet longer.

It is hoped that no one who recovers from his or her problem by following the Specific Carbohydrate Diet ever returns to a diet high in refined sugar and refined flours. These are lacking or low in nutrients, will not nourish the immunological system adequately, and can make the individual more susceptible to intestinal infections. We kept our child on the diet for seven years although the symptoms had disappeared at the end of two. We enjoyed this way of eating and preferred to be cautious. Since Dr.Haas had died two years after the diet was initiated, we had no way of knowing the right time to go off the diet and, realizing how highly nutritious the diet was, we decided not to risk going off it too soon.

Chapter 8

THE SPECIFIC CARBOHYDRATE DIET

ALLOWABLE PROTEINS (Meat, fish, dairy products, etc.)
All fresh or frozen beef, lamb, pork, poultry, fish (including shellfish), eggs, natural cheeses (listed in Appendix), homemade yoghurt made according to recipe in Gourmet Section, **DRY CURD** cottage cheese. Canned fish (canned in oil or water).

NOT PERMITTED
Processed meats such as hot dogs, bologna, turkey loaf, spiced ham, breaded fish, canned fish with sauces, processed cheeses (listed in Appendix), smoked meats (unless you know definitely that sugar has not been added at some stage in the smoking process). Most available smoked meats contain considerable amounts of refined sugar. In many parts of the country, abattoirs are available that will smoke meats according to your specifications. However, for those people who cannot get their meat smoked without sugar, ordinary smoked bacon may be eaten once a week if it is fried very crisply.
Most processed meats are not permitted since they contain starch, whey powder, lactose, or sucrose. It may be possible to obtain hot dogs and other processed meats without these additives and, if so, they may be included in the diet. NO CANNED MEATS PERMITTED.

ALLOWABLE VEGETABLES - Fresh or frozen (with no added sugar or starch). NO CANNED VEGETABLES PERMITTED.
Artichoke (French but not Jerusalem), asparagus, beets, dried white (navy) beans, lentils, and split peas (dried

legumes prepared according to instructions in Gourmet Section), broccoli, brussell sprouts, cabbage, cauliflower, carrots, celery, cucumbers, eggplant, garlic, kale, lettuce of all kinds, lima beans (dried and fresh), mushrooms, onions, parsley, peas, pumpkin, spinach, squash (summer and winter), string beans, tomatoes, turnips, watercress.

Snacks can include raw vegetables provided that diarrhea is not active.

NOT PERMITTED
Grains such as wheat, barley, corn, rye, oats, rice, buckwheat, millet, triticale, bulgur. (No cereals or flour made from these).
Potatoes (white or sweet), yams, parsnips.
Chick peas, bean sprouts, soybeans, mungbeans, faba beans, garbanzo beans.
Amaranth flour, quinoa flour, or any newly-introduced grain substitutes such as cottonseed.
Wheat germ. Seaweeds.
Caution: Many recipes from other countries, such as cous-cous, contain grain-like ingredients which must be avoided.

ALLOWABLE FRUITS - Fresh, raw or cooked, frozen (with no added sugar), and dried. Canned fruits which state ''canned in own juice''; none canned in any other kind of juice. In sweetening cooked or raw fruits, use honey or saccharin. No other artificial sweetener but saccharin is allowed.

Apples, avocadoes, apricots, bananas (ripe with black spots beginning to appear on skin), berries of all kinds (including blueberries), cherries, fresh coconut or unsweetened shredded coconut, dates (only loose California dates are permitted; dates which stick together in a mass have had syrup or sugar added and are not permitted), grapefruit, grapes, Kiwi fruit, kumquats, lemons, limes, mangoes, melons, nectarines, oranges, papayas, peaches, pears, pineapples (glazed pineapple is permitted only if the glaze is the result of the drying of the natural sugars in the pineapple), prunes, raisins (preferably dark), rhubarb. tangerines.

Some people are allergic to sulfites and should avoid dried fruit to which these have been added. If there is no sensitivity to sulfites, this type of dried fruit may be used occasionally.

Dried banana chips are usually coated with corn syrup or refined sugar and should be avoided unless they are known to be produced without such additives.

ALLOWABLE NUTS - Purchased with or without shells.

Almonds, pecans, Brazil nuts, filberts (hazelnuts), walnuts, unroasted cashews, chestnuts. Peanut butter, without additives of any kind. Roasted peanuts in the shell may be tried cautiously after being on the diet about six months when diarrhea is gone. Avoid shelled peanuts as most have added starch. Nuts sold in salted mixtures are not permissable since most have been roasted with a starch coating.

ALLOWABLE BEVERAGES (See Appendix)
JUICES

Canned tomato juice and V-8 are permissible (only salt added).

Use tomato juice for cooking *instead* of canned tomato paste, canned tomato sauce, or canned tomato puréc. Avoid canned tomato juice mixtures such as tomato juice cocktail or other tomato juice mixtures.

Orange juice, fresh, frozen without added sugar, and canned orange and grapefruit juices without added sugar. While diarrhea is active, AVOID ORANGE JUICE IN THE MORNING. If taken in the morning, it tends to increase diarrhea. However, it appears to be well tolerated later in the day.

Grape juice, white or dark. Bottled grape juice usually has no added sugar; avoid frozen grape juice which usually does have added sugar.

Pineapple juice (canned, frozen, or fresh) without added sugar.

Apple juice, formerly an allowable beverage, has become a problem because some manufacturers are adding corn syrup and sugar which is not listed on the label.

Therefore, choose an apple *cider* packed by a local company you feel is responsible. You can call or write to them to ensure that it is pure apple cider without added sweetener. A preservative such as sodium benzoate is permissible. It is still possible in many areas to obtain freshly pressed apple cider and freeze enough for a year (Caution: fill containers only two-thirds full).

Juices packed in boxes, even those which state that there has been no sugar added, should be avoided since experience has shown that they are not well tolerated by those on the Specific Carbohydrate Diet.

Freshly squeezed vegetable juices of any of the allowed vegetables.

OTHER BEVERAGES

Weak tea or very weak coffee, perked or dripped, without milk or cream.

Ground chickory may be added to perked or dripped coffee to give a stronger flavor.

Some herb teas can be laxative. Restrict the use of herb teas to peppermint and spearmint.

Milkshakes made with homemade yoghurt, fruits, sweetened to taste with honey or saccharin.

NOT PERMITTED
Fluid milk of any kind.
Dried milk solids.
Commercially prepared acidophilus milk which contains unfermented milk along with the acidophilus bacteria; much lactose remains.
Commercial buttermilk, commercial sour cream, or commercial yoghurt (except for use as a starter for your own homemade yoghurt). Some companies are producing sour cream which contains virtually no lactose. Inquire concerning the availability of this permissible product in your area.
Enzyme-treated milk, except as noted in Chapter 7; milk drunk along with lactase enzyme replacement (in vivo replacement).

Soybean milk.

Instant tea or coffee.

Coffee substitutes; most have malt added which is not permitted.

Postum.

ALLOWABLE CONFECTIONS

A person on the Specific Carbohydrate Diet does not have to be denied sweets and other confections. With the use of honey, nuts, dried fruits, the most delicious cakes, cookies, muffins, and candies may be made.

ADDITIONAL INSTRUCTIONS

Although grains are not permitted, salad and cooking oils made from grains may be used; therefore, corn and soybean oils are permitted. Other oils which may be used for salads and cooking are sunflower and safflower oils. Olive oil is highly recommended.

Thicken gravy with boiled onion puréed in blender or with homemade mayonnaise (see Gourmet Section for gravy).

Unflavored gelatin is to be used for gelatin-type desserts.

Mustard is permissible; use plain mustard since gourmet types have many added ingredients which must be avoided.

Dill pickles and olives are permissible. Read labels carefully and avoid those with added sugar.

Vinegar is permitted (cider or white). Some gourmet-type vinegars have added sugar and should not be used.

Diet soft drinks are permitted occasionally. Those sweetened with aspartame or Nutri-Sweet may sometimes contain lactose and should be avoided, if possible. However, if this is the only type available, one per week is permitted. Diet soft drinks sweetened with saccharin need not be limited to only one a week: 2-3 weekly would be permissible. If the soft drink **specifically** states that it is sweetened with fructose or glucose, (monosaccharide sugars) or a combination of both, 2-3 weekly are permissible.

Use butter, not margarine. Margarine contains added milk solids and/or whey.

Whey butter may be used since it contains only the fat extracted from the whey and not the lactose.

Spices of all kinds may be used. Avoid mixtures such as "apple pie spices" and curry powder; buy spices such as cinnamon and nutmeg separately.

Use fresh garlic and onions instead of garlic and onion powders which may have a starch base.

Coconut milk and almond milk may be tried after six months.

Pasta such as spaghetti and macaroni is made from grains and is forbidden. There are substitutes for pizza and spaghetti in the Gourmet Section.

Do not use cornstarch, arrowroot starch, tapioca starch, sago starch, or other starches of any kind.

Do not use chocolate or carob.

Do not use bouillon cubes or instant soup bases.

DO NOT USE PRODUCTS MADE WITH REFINED SUGAR. This eliminates many commercially prepared products, some of which are listed in the Appendix.

Do not use agar-agar or carrageenan.

Do not use pectin in making jellies and jams (see recipes for jams in Gourmet Section).

Ketchup is almost 40% sugar and is not permissible. (see Gourmet Section for a quick ketchup).

No ice cream unless you make your own. Commercial ice cream is very high in lactose and sucrose. Even those commercial ice creams made with honey are often high in lactose.

No molasses, corn syrup, or maple syrup.

Do not use flours made from beans or lentils since beans and lentils were probably not soaked prior to grinding. If they are marked "presoaked," the flour may be used sparingly. Soaked and cooked navy beans (see instructions in Gourmet Section) may be drained and puréed and used in some of the cake recipes as an "extender" in order to cut back on the quantity of nut flour required.

Do not use baking powder. Use baking soda where specified.

Do not use seeds of any kind until three months after the last symptom has disappeared and then try them cautiously.

Although all natural cheeses may be used (see Appendix), there are two cheeses which are considered natural which must be avoided. They are Ricotta and Mozarella. The brown, carmelized cheese called Gjetost must also be avoided.

Many medications have added sugars of the wrong kind (sucrose and lactose). Some of these medications may be obtained without these sugars by asking your pharmacist. Glucose (dextrose) or fructose (levulose) are permitted additives.

ALCOHOLIC BEVERAGES

Avoid beer.

Very dry wine is permissible. If a sweeter wine is desired, add a crushed saccharin tablet or sweeten with honey.

Occasionally gin, rye, Scotch, bourbon, vodka, etc. No sherry, cordials, liqueurs, or brandy.

Club soda is permissible as a mixer since it has no added sugar.

The following is a sample day's menu. The quantity of foods eaten should depend upon appetite. It is presented to give an idea of how the Specific Carbohydrate Diet can be implemented.

BREAKFAST
Baked apple sweetened with honey, if desired; cinnamon to flavor
Scrambled eggs
Homemade nut muffin with butter and homemade jam
Weak tea, coffee, grape juice, or apple cider

LUNCH
Tuna fish salad made with homemade mayonnaise, garnished with olives, dill pickle, on a bed of lettuce
Slices of cheddar cheese
Homemade pumpkin pie (recipe in Gourmet Section)
         Nut crust can be used or the filling can be eaten as a pudding
Piña Colada made according to recipe in Gourmet Section

DINNER
Homemade spaghetti sauce made with ground beef, onions, garlic, herbs, tomato juice. Serve on a bed of boiled beans or spaghetti squash
Freshly grated cabbage salad with homemade mayonnaise or oil and vinegar
Peas and carrots with butter
Fresh fruit or cheese cake (recipe in Gourmet Section)
Tea

GOURMET SECTION

TABLE OF CONTENTS

MAIN DISHES, POULTRY STUFFING, GRAVY

MUFFINS, BREAD, AND PANCAKES

CAKES

FROSTINGS

COOKIES

DESSERTS

SWEET TREATS, JAM

BEVERAGES

MILK PREPARATIONS AND INFANT FORMULA

APPETIZERS, DIPS, AND SPREADS

Apple-Raisin Peanut Butter Spread

This spread may be used on slices of cheddar cheese or as a dip.

½ cup peanut butter
(no additives)
½ cup unpeeled, diced apple

¼ cup raisins
½ teaspoon ground
cinnamon

In a small bowl stir together peanut butter, apple, raisins, and cinnamon.
If too stiff to spread, add a little apple cider and blend ingredients together.

Liver Paté

1 lb. tender liver
(chicken or calf)
¼-½ cup homemade
mayonnaise (see pg.69)

1 small onion, cut into
small pieces
salt and pepper to taste

Pan fry liver in butter until it has lost its pink color.
Cool liver and cut into small pieces.
Place liver, onion, and mayonnaise in blender or food processor.
(If using blender, place mayonnaise at bottom so that blades will turn easily.)
Blend until smooth.
Serve as a stuffing for celery, on lettuce leaves, or as a dip with raw vegetables.
Can be spread on squares of cheese and served as an appetizer.

Party Cheese Dip

*1 ½ cups cheddar cheese,
  grated*
¼ cup soft butter
*¼ teaspoon dry mustard
  powder*

*⅓ cup apple cider or dry
  white wine*
*fruits such as apple or
  pear wedges or raw
  vegetables*

Cream the butter; blend in mustard powder and cider.
Add the grated cheese and blend thoroughly.
Chill overnight, if possible, to blend flavors.
Allow to stand at room temperature for ½-1 hour.
Use with fruits or vegetables.

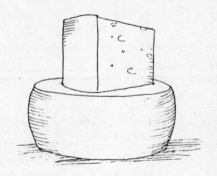

SOUPS

Carrot Soup

*2 lbs. carrots, scrubbed and
 quartered lengthwise*
*4 cups homemade chicken
 stock*
1 cup finely chopped onion

*2 small cloves garlic,
 crushed*
1 cup homemade yoghurt
⅓ cup chopped almonds
3-4 tablespoons butter

Salt chicken stock to taste
Parboil carrots in chicken stock about 12-15 minutes. Cool.
Sauté the onion, garlic, and chopped almonds in 3-4 tablespoons butter until tender but not browned.
Purée carrots, stock, sautéed mixture, and yoghurt in a blender until smooth.
Add seasoning of your choice†.
Heat very slowly in a double boiler or chill and serve cold.
Garnish with toasted nuts, parsley or cress.

† Suggested seasoning combinations from which to choose:
1. pinch nutmeg, ½ teaspoon mint, dash of cinnamon, OR
2. ½-1 teaspoon thyme, ½-1 teaspoon marjoram, ½-1 teaspoon basil, OR
3. 1 teaspoon freshly grated ginger root sautéed in butter.

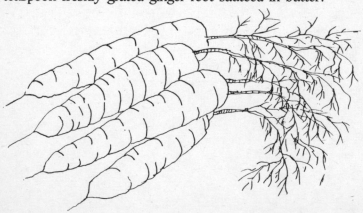

Cream of Tomato Soup

2 cups tomato juice
½-1 cup homemade yoghurt
(see pg.115)

honey or saccharin to
taste

Make a paste with the yoghurt and ¼ cup tomato juice.
Slowly stir in the remaining juice.
Heat over low heat or in a double boiler, stirring occasionally.
Season to taste with salt, pepper, sweetener, and herbs of choice.

Gazpacho Soup

4 cups tomato juice
1 small well-minced onion
2 cups diced fresh tomatoes
1 cup minced green pepper
1 cup diced medium
  cucumber (peeled)
1 clove garlic, crushed
juice of ½ lemon

juice of 1 lime (optional)
2 tablespoons white vinegar
1 teaspoon tarragon
  (optional)
1 teaspoon basil
¼ cup freshly chopped
  parsley
2 tablespoons olive oil
salt and pepper to taste

Garnish: 1 hard boiled egg yolk chopped with a little parsley (optional)

Combine all ingredients.
Chill for at least two hours before serving.
Note: Ingredients may be processed in a blender instead of chopping separately.

Hearty Vegetable Soup

1 cup chopped celery
1 cup chopped carrots
1 cup chopped onion
½ cup chopped cabbage
2 cups tomato juice or a few
fresh tomatoes
2 cups homemade chicken
or beef stock OR

4 cups water and about 1
lb. beef bones (or ½-1 lb.
beef)
2 tablespoons oil or butter
Season to taste (herbs and
spices such as basil, salt,
pepper, bay leaf)

If a food processor is available, all vegetables may be chopped in a few minutes using the steel blade.

Sauté onions and carrots in oil or butter until soft.

Add all other ingredients and simmer for 2 hours if stock is used; for 3-4 hours if beef bones or beef is used.

Chicken Soup

Using the largest pot you have, fill half of it with chicken parts (legs and thighs make the most flavorful soup).

Peel about ten carrots and add to chicken.

Add about two large onions, a few stalks of celery, and some parsley.

Season with salt.

Fill pot with water.

Simmer for about 4 hours and then strain soup through a colander or strainer.

Purée carrots in blender and return to broth.

Remove skin from chicken parts and return to broth.

Onions, celery, and parsley should not be used at the start of the dietary regimen because the fibrous parts of these vegetables may cause problems.

CONDIMENTS, SALADS, AND SALAD DRESSINGS

CONDIMENTS

Chili Sauce

*1 - 6 qt. basket ripe
tomatoes, unpeeled,
chopped
6 cups celery, chopped
4 cups onions, chopped*

*2 cups green peppers,
chopped
2½ cups vinegar
1 tablespoon salt
3 cups honey
dash of pepper*

All ingredients may be chopped very quickly in a food processor.
Combine all ingredients.
Bring to a boil in a large pot, stirring more often as the chili sauce
thickens. STIR FREQUENTLY to prevent scorching.
Simmer for about 30 minutes depending upon thickness desired.
Cool. Pack in plastic containers and freeze OR bottle and seal.

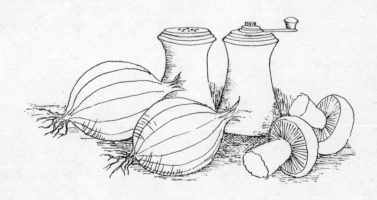

Honey-Ginger Chutney

1¼ cups honey
1 cup cider vinegar
6 or 7 cooking apples
2 lemons
2 green peppers or sweet
   red peppers
3 medium onions

1½ cups canned crushed
   unsweetened pineapple,
   including juice
1 cup raisins
4 teaspoons fresh ginger,
   grated
¾ cup almonds, slivered

Heat the honey and vinegar in a large saucepan.
Peel, core, and dice apples finely.
Add apples to the honey and vinegar and simmer for 20 minutes.
Remove the seeds and chop peppers and lemons finely, preferably in a food processor using the metal blade, and add to apple mixture.
Stir in the finely chopped onions.
Add the pineapple, raisins and ginger.
Simmer for 20 minutes more.
Add the slivered almonds and simmer for 30 minutes; stir frequently to prevent sticking.

Ketchup

2 cups tomato juice
1-3 tablespoons white
   vinegar
honey and/or saccharin to
   taste

bay leaf (optional)
salt and pepper to taste

Mix all ingredients except sweetener and simmer on stove until thick, stirring often to prevent sticking.
When almost the desired thickness, add sweetener to taste and complete cooking.
Ladle into sterilized jars and seal immediately OR place in small containers and freeze.

Raw Cranberry Relish

1 lb. fresh cranberries   *1 apple*
1 orange   *honey*

Wash and drain cranberries.

Cut orange into small pieces and remove seeds (orange need not be peeled).

Core apple and cut into small pieces.

Combine ingredients and process using blender, processor, or hand grinder until well mixed.

Sweeten to taste with honey.

Serve with meat or poultry or mix with dry curd uncreamed cottage cheese and serve on lettuce.

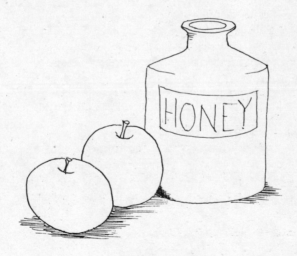

SALADS

Cottage Cheese Salad

*1 cup uncreamed cottage
    cheese (dry white curd)*
¼ cup homemade yoghurt

*¼ cup unsweetened
    pineapple (fresh or
    canned) or other fruit in
    season*

Mix ingredients together and serve on lettuce.

Halloween Carrot Salad (Pumpkin Heads)

2 cups grated raw carrots
*½ cup homemade
    mayonnaise*

lettuce leaves

Garnish: a few dark raisins and strips of green pepper

Mix carrots with mayonnaise.
Fill a small cup with carrot salad and unmold onto a lettuce-covered plate.
Make eyes and nose of pumpkin head using raisins.
Use strip of green pepper for mouth.

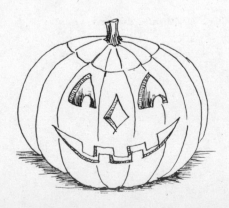

Mock Antipasto Salad

1 can anchovies
1 or 2 hard boiled eggs,
    quartered
2 fresh tomatoes, diced or
    sliced

lettuce, shredded
Italian herbs (oregano,
    basil), if desired
Oil and vinegar dressing

Mix all ingredients and chill.

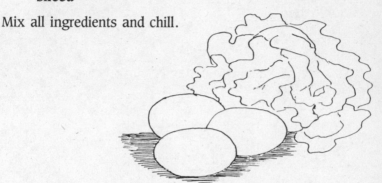

Seafood Salad

1 can tuna, salmon, or
    crabmeat or 1 lb. cooked
    and chilled bland fish
    (sole, halibut, cod, etc.)

½ cup homemade
    mayonnaise
lettuce leaves

Drain oil or water from canned fish.
Flake fish with a fork.
Add as much mayonnaise as desired, mix thoroughly, and chill.
Heap onto a bed of lettuce.

Waldorf Salad

*3 cups apples, cut in chunks
   or ½ inch cubes (peeled
   or unpeeled)
1 cup pineapple chunks
   (fresh or canned,
   unsweetened)
¼ cup raisins*

*1 stalk celery, chopped
½ cup thinly-sliced green
   pepper (optional)
1 cup thinly-sliced raw
   carrots (optional)
¼-½ cup walnut pieces*

Combine all ingredients.
Blend with 1 cup of yoghurt dressing or mayonnaise.
Serve on lettuce leaves.

Zucchini and Tomato Salad

*2 cups diced uncooked
   zucchini or cucumber
2 cups diced fresh tomatoes
   (include juice)
¼ cup chopped green onion*

*1 small green pepper cut
   into narrow ribbons
1 stalk celery, chopped
vinaigrette dressing*

Prepare vegetables and add dressing.
Chill in refrigerator for one hour before serving.

SALAD DRESSINGS

Mayonnaise

May be made in a blender or food processor (using steel blade).
If made in processor, recipe can be doubled. However, the recipe cannot be doubled if a blender is used; it will not thicken properly.

1 whole egg
1-1¼ cups oil
1 tablespoon white vinegar
*   or fresh lemon juice*
¼ teaspoon dry mustard
*   powder*

salt and pepper to taste
1 crushed saccharin
*   (¼ grain)*
or a little honey
(optional)

Any vegetable oil or a combination of oils may be used.
Process in blender or processor for a few seconds: egg, lemon juice (or vinegar), and mustard.
While the machine is running, add the oil in a fine stream.
Do not add oil quickly; it should take at least 60 seconds.
As mayonnaise thickens, the sound of the machine will deepen.

Suggestions:
Use to thicken gravy: Add 2 tablespoons mayonnaise to about 1 cup
    of gravy liquid and heat gently for about 1-2 minutes, stirring
    constantly.
Use as a base for tartar sauce by adding ½ cup chopped dill pickles
    (unsweetened) and ¼ chopped onion.
Use as a mock Hollandaise sauce by adding grated cheddar cheese:
    Spread on vegetables such as cooked cauliflower or broccoli.
    Cover and heat in oven.
Mix with yoghurt (1 part mayonnaise, 1 part homemade yoghurt) and
    use as a salad dressing.

Vinaigrette Dressing

May be used for salads or for marinating chilled vegetables
Combine in a small bowl:

¼ teaspoon salt
¼ teaspoon pepper
1 tablespoon olive oil

1 tablespoon vinegar or
lemon juice
¼ teaspoon dry mustard
powder

Beat these ingredients well with a fork or a wisk until blended.
Add:

1 tablespoon vinegar or
lemon juice

3 tablespoons olive oil
1 whole clove garlic, peeled

Store in a covered jar in a cold place until ready for use.
Shake well before using.

Yoghurt Salad Dressing

May be used for fruit salads or vegetable salads

1 cup homemade yoghurt
Juice of 1 lemon
honey or crushed saccharin

Mix yoghurt and lemon juice and sweeten to taste with liquid honey
or crushed saccharin tablets.

VEGETABLES

Baked Acorn (Pepper) Squash

1 acorn squash
a little butter
a little honey

grated orange rind
(¼ teaspoon for each
squash half)

Cut acorn squash in half and use ½ squash for each serving
Scoop out seed cavity of each squash half.
Place cut side down on a cookie sheet and bake at 400° F. (200° C.)
until a dull knife goes through squash easily.
Turn face up and dot with butter, honey, and grated orange rind.
Return to oven and bake another 15-30 minutes at 350° F. (180° C.).

Variation: These squash "boats" may also be filled with a mixture
of cooked poultry or cooked meat which has been mixed with vegetables
and moistened with broth, yoghurt, or onion gravy (see pg.77).

Butternut Squash Slices

1 butternut squash
small amount butter
salt to taste

Slice the neck of a butternut squash (not necessary to peel). If crispness
is desired, slice very thinly, about ¼ inch thick. If cut thinly, these
may be used as a substitute for french-fried potatoes.
Place on cookie sheet or pizza pan, dot with butter, and bake in a hot
oven 450° F. (230° C.). until one side is brown.
Turn and brown other side.

Carrot Curls

This recipe may be used as a substitute for potato chips or when something crisp is desired.
Using a potato peeler, make curls out of about 3 carrots.
Deep fry in oil until they turn golden brown.
Drain in a colander or strainer. Refrigerate oil for next batch.
(Do not use oil more than 3 times as it may become rancid.)
Turn carrot curls onto a paper towel and pat dry.
Salt to taste.

Cauliflower "Potatoes"

This a delicious substitute for mashed potatoes.

1 large cauliflower, cut into pieces
¼ cup butter or ¼ cup homemade yoghurt

salt, pepper to taste
parsley and paprika garnish

Cook cauliflower until just tender. Drain.
Purée in blender or food processor.
Add butter or yoghurt, salt and pepper, and blend thoroughly.
Reheat and serve.
Garnish with parsley and paprika.
The puréed cauliflower may be placed in a baking dish, sprinkled with grated cheddar cheese and heated in the oven until the cheese melts.

French Fried Turnips (Rutabagas)

1 medium-sized yellow
turnip, peeled
⅓ cup vegetable oil

Cut turnip into pieces the size of french fries.
Pour oil into large pan and place cut turnip pieces into pan.
Rub oil over surfaces of turnip pieces.
Bake in hot oven 400° F. (200° C.) for about 1 hour or until turnips
are well browned and cooked through.

(Recipe courtesy of May Rodall)

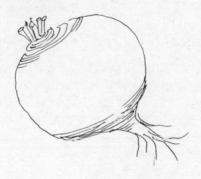

Sweet and Sour Lentils

1 cup lentils   *3 tablespoons honey*
2 tablespoons white vinegar   *2 tablespoons butter*

Soak lentils overnight and throw away the water.
Add fresh water to cover lentils and simmer until tender. Drain.
Add remaining ingredients, heat and serve.

MAIN DISHES, POULTRY STUFFING, GRAVY

Baked Bean Casserole

Introduce this recipe after being on the diet for at least 3 months.

1 lb. dried white beans
1-2 whole onions
meaty bone (ham, beef,
etc.)
1 large can tomato juice (48
fluid ounces)

½-1 teaspoon dry mustard
powder
3 tablespoons vinegar
3-6 tablespoons honey
salt and pepper

Soak beans overnight in cold water. Drain and throw away water. Rinse beans thoroughly under running water.
Cover with fresh water and simmer at low heat until beans are tender. This may take over 2 hours. Do not salt beans before boiling; they will not become tender.
Add remaining ingredients and bake in oven at 300° F. (150° C.) until beans are very soft and tomato juice has thickened.
More tomato juice may have to be added while beans are baking to prevent them from sticking to the pan and burning.
Stir occasionally.
Beans should bake a minimum of 2 hours.
Before serving, cut meat off bone and discard bone.
Serve hot or cold.

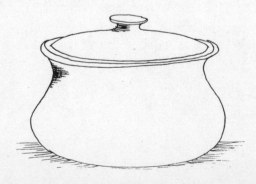

Baked Cottage Cheese

1 cup uncreamed cottage cheese (dry curd)	*1 teaspoon honey*
	1 teaspoon butter
1 egg	

Blend all ingredients.
Pour mixture into a greased baking dish and bake at 350° F. (180° C.) until of firm consistency and slighty browned around the edges (about 15 or 20 minutes).

Chicken Royale

2 lbs. chicken parts	*2 whole green onions, including stems, sliced*
1 cup sliced or diced carrots	
1 cup fresh or frozen cauliflower pieces	*4 cloves fresh garlic*
	1 tablespoon oil
1 whole tomato, diced	*½ teaspoon paprika*
	salt to taste

Wash and drain chicken parts.
Heat oil, add garlic and green onions and sauté for 2 minutes.
Add chicken and cook for 5 minutes.
Add paprika and tomato, cover and cook for 10 minutes on medium heat.
Add cauliflower, carrots, and salt and cook for antother 5 minutes.

(Recipe courtesy of Zairun and Aleesa Hosein)

Fish Casserole

*1 lb. fresh, frozen, or
canned fish (halibut,
flounder, sole, shrimp,
lobster, or crabmeat)
½ lb. grated cheddar cheese
1 cup homemade yoghurt*

*1 teaspoon dry mustard
powder
1 tablespoon chopped
parsley
1 tablespoon lemon juice*

Poach fresh or frozen fish for a few minutes until cooked through.
Drain, if using canned fish, or cool poached fish and, using fork, break
into bite-size pieces.
Mix remaining ingredients thoroughly and add to fish.
Bake in ovenware at 375° F. (190° C.) until brown on top. This should
take about 30-40 minutes.
This recipe may also be used as an appetizer. Bake as instructed and
serve in small portions.

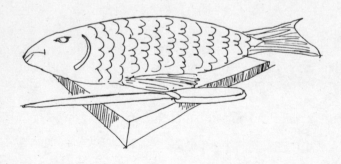

Ginger-Yoghurt Chicken

4 whole chicken breasts
2 cups homemade yoghurt
½ cup nut flour (see
   Basic Muffin Recipe,
   pg.87 for preparation of
   flour)

1 teaspoon freshly grated
   ginger
salt to taste
butter for frying chicken

Split each breast down the back into two pieces.
Heat frying pan, add butter and brown the raw chicken. Do not cook completely.
Salt chicken.
Remove from heat.
Mix yoghurt, almond flour, and grated ginger.
Arrange chicken in a single layer in an oven-safe pan.
Spread the yoghurt mixture over the surface of each piece of chicken, using all of the mixture.
Place, uncovered, in a 325° F. (160° C.) oven.
Bake ½ hour or until chicken is tender.

(Recipe courtesy of Zairun Hosein)

Gravy

May be used as a thickened gravy for poultry or meat.

Type 1:
While roast is in the oven, boil an onion.
While poultry is in oven, boil an onion together with poultry giblets.
When the meat is done, pour the drippings into a container and skim off fat.
Place cooked onion and skimmed drippings (at least 1 cup) into blender and purée.

Type 2:
For each cup of liquid, add 2 tablespoons of homemade mayonnaise.
Heat gently for about a minute, stirring constantly.

(Recipe courtesy of Roberta Young)

Honey-Garlic Chicken Wings

2 lbs. chicken wings
1 tablespoon butter
¼ cup honey
1 teaspoon grated lemon
   rind

1 tablespoon lemon juice
salt and pepper to taste
crushed garlic clove

Place wings in baking dish.
Melt butter and add honey, lemon juice and rind.
Dust wings with salt and pepper.
Pour half of honey mixture over wings and coat evenly.
Bake wings at 350° F. (180° C.) for 15 minutes.
Add remaining honey mixture.
Continue baking until wings are tender and browned.

Honey-Garlic Spareribs

3 lbs. pork spareribs or ham
   hocks (unsmoked)
½ cup honey
1 cup water

2-4 tablespoons crushed
   fresh garlic or 4
   tablespoons garlic chips
1 teaspoon salt

Parboil pork and remove excess fat if hocks are used.
Mix remaining ingredients and pour over parboiled pork which has been
placed in a large roasting pan or baking dish.
Bake at 375° F. (190° C.) for at least 1 hour turning and basting at
least twice until the honey begins to carmelize on the meat.

Pizza

Crust:

3½ cups coarsely grated,
  unpeeled, zucchini
  squash†

3 eggs, lightly beaten

⅓ cup almond flour

½ cup grated brick cheese
  (any permissible mild
  cheese will do)

½ cup grated, 100% pure,
  parmesan cheese

1 tablespoon fresh basil
  leaves, minced (dried
  may be substituted but
  use only about
  ¼ tablespoon)

¼ teaspoon salt

†Salt grated zucchini squash with ¼ teaspoon salt and let stand for 15 minutes to draw out excess water. Squeeze zucchini with hands to get rid of as much water as possible.

Mix all ingredients well and spread onto an oiled pizza pan or small cookie sheet. Pat smooth.

Bake for 30 minutes at 325° F. (160° C.) or until crust is dry and browned.

Brush the top of the crust with oil and broil it under moderate heat for 5 minutes.

Alternative crust recipe: Cheese bread recipe (pg. 89) may be used. For a large pizza, use about ⅓ of recipe. Pat down in pizza pan until about ⅓ - ½" thick. Bake at 350 deg. F. until golden brown and proceed by adding filling.

Filling:

½-1 lb. brick cheese, thinly
  sliced

1½ cups tomato sauce
  (made by simmering
  about 3-4 cups tomato
  juice)

a few of the following:
  mushrooms, olives, strips of
  green pepper, crisply
  fried bacon pieces,
  cooked ham slivers,
  anchovies, tomato slices,
  etc.

Layer cheese on baked crust.

Spread generously with thick tomato sauce.

Add your choice of toppings.

Heat pizza in a 350° F. (180° C.) oven for about 25 minutes until it is very hot and cheese is bubbling.

Serve hot with a tossed salad.

Poultry Stuffing
(For a large bird)

2 cups dried white beans   *1 teaspoon ground sage*
  (navy beans)   *1 teaspoon ground thyme*
1 cup chopped onion   *chopped parsley (optional)*
½ cup chopped celery   *salt and pepper to taste*

Soak beans overnight and throw away the water.
Cover with fresh water (do not salt before cooking or beans will be tough) and cook until tender. Drain.
Mix chopped onion, celery, and herbs with beans and mash with a potato masher.
Season to taste with salt and pepper.
Fill cavity of turkey or chicken with bean mixture and roast.

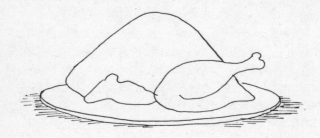

"Spaghetti" and Sauce

1 lb. ground beef (lean)
1 large can tomato juice (48
    fluid ounces)
3-4 fresh tomatoes, if
    available
1 large onion
1-2 cloves garlic (optional)
1 bay leaf

½-1 teaspoon oregano
1 tablespoon olive oil
salt and pepper to taste
1 spaghetti squash (most
    large supermarkets can
    get these if they don't
    carry them)

Sauce:

Chop onion and garlic and brown in oil in a heavy skillet.

Remove onion, set aside, and brown meat in the same pan.

Transfer meat and onion to large pot and add tomato juice, bay leaf, oregano and seasonings.

Simmer to desired thickeness; this may take 1 hour or longer.

Spaghetti Squash:

Cut the spaghetti squash in half lengthwise.

Steam on a rack over boiling water in a large covered pan or steamer until just tender. DO NOT overcook as squash can become too soft and watery.

Lift out strings of "spaghetti" from squash with a fork.

Serve smothered in hot spaghetti sauce.

Grated parmesan or romano cheese may be used to top.

The spaghetti sauce may also be used to top boiled white (navy) beans or another type of squash (zucchini, butternut, hubbard).

Stir-Fried Vegetables with Chicken, Beef, or Pork

cauliflower pieces
broccoli pieces, including
  the stem
celery, sliced
carrots, sliced
zucchini squash, sliced
mushrooms, sliced
tomatoes, quartered

peppers, sliced in strips
onions, sliced
edible-podded peas
  (optional)
chicken breasts, steamed OR
  sirloin or round steak,
  semi-frozen

The quantity of each ingredient depends on the number-of people to be served.
A heavy iron frying pan or a wok should be used.
Sauté in butter, using medium heat, any combination of, or all of, the listed vegetables.
Begin by cooking the vegetables that take longer to tenderize (carrots, cauliflower, broccoli).
After a few minutes, add the rest of the vegetables, except the tomatoes.
Turn heat to simmer, cover pan or wok, and cook until all vegetables are barely tender.
Add tomatoes and cook about 1 minute longer.
Season with salt and pepper.
Add prepared meat or chicken and serve piping hot.

Preparation of meat:
Chicken: Steam until tender. Remove skin and bones. Cut in large chunks. Brown in a separate pan in butter. A little honey may be added to the meat if desired. Set aside until you are ready to combine with vegetables.
Beef: Semi-frozen beef is easy to slice. Slice in thin strips, across grain. Brown pieces of beef in a separate skillet in butter. Set aside until ready to combine with vegetables.
Pork: Use left-over pork roast. Slice in thin strips and set aside until ready to combine with vegetables.

Stuffed Zucchini

6 zucchini squash
1 garlic clove, crushed
1½ cups ground beef
1 cup cheddar cheese (or other hard cheese), grated

2 eggs slightly beaten
4 tablespoons melted butter
salt and pepper to taste
1 tablespoon chopped fresh basil or ¼ teaspoon dried basil (optional)

Pan fry the ground beef in a little butter until cooked through.
Cut the zucchini squash in half lengthwise and carefully hollow out the flesh to within ¼ inch of the skin.
Set the shells aside.
Chop the zucchini flesh, then press with the back of a wooden spoon to extract as much juice as possible and drain it away.
Set the flesh aside.
Preheat oven to 400° F. (200° C.)
Combine the zucchini flesh, garlic, ground beef, basil, cheese, seasoning, eggs and half the melted butter until they are thoroughly blended.
Arrange the zucchini shells skin-side down in a well-greased shallow baking pan.
Stuff with the beef mixture and pour the remaining melted butter over the stuffed squash.
Place dish in oven and bake for 20-30 minutes or until the top is brown and bubbling.
Serve at once.

Vegetable Meat Loaf

1 ½ lbs. ground beef
1 egg
1 medium fresh tomato or
    ½ cup tomato juice
1 medium onion, cut in
    pieces

sprig of parsley
1 stalk of celery, cut in
    pieces
small amount of green
    pepper
1 carrot, cut in pieces

Place tomato or tomato juice into blender first. Push down on tomato to release juices so that blender blades will turn easily.

Add egg and blend for a few seconds.

Add remaining vegetables and blend until fairly smooth.†

Empty blender contents into bowl and mix well with ground beef.

Season with salt and pepper.

Form mixture into a loaf and place in a shallow pan.

Spread top with homemade quick ketchup (see pg.64).

Bake in 350° F. (180° C.) oven for about 1 hour.

†You may have to stop blender and push vegetables down in order for them to make contact with blender blades.

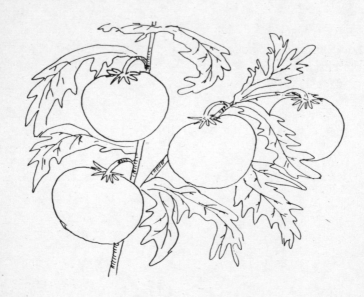

Zucchini Casserole

Use any amount of the vegetables specified; the size of your pan or casserole should be your guide.

zucchini squash, sliced
fresh tomatoes, sliced
onions, sliced
green peppers, sliced
   (optional)
1 tablespoon salad oil
   (olive oil is best in this
recipe) for each 4 cups of
vegetables
½ cup grated Parmesan
   cheese (optional)
Seasonings: oregano, salt,
   pepper

Slice raw vegetables and layer in a casserole. A shallow casserole is preferable but any size may be used.

Pour salad oil over vegetables.

Sprinkle seasonings and grated cheese over top.

Add a little water to casserole if there is not sufficient juices from the vegetables. There should be at least ½ inch liquid at the bottom of the casserole when you start baking.

Place in hot oven 400° F. (200° C.), uncovered, and bake until vegetables are tender.

Stir occasionally so that the top vegetables do not get too brown.

If this recipe is made on top of stove, it turns out to be a vegetable stew and has a completely different consistency.

Zucchini Lasagna

1½ lbs. ground beef
2 medium-sized zucchini
    squash, cut lengthwise in
    ½ inch slices
2 cups uncreamed cottage
    cheese (dry curd)
1 cup tomato juice
½ cup colby, brick, or
havarti cheese, grated or
    sliced for topping.
1 medium-sized onion
1 cup mushrooms, sliced
    (optional)
1 teaspoon oregano
¼ teaspoon ground basil
salt and pepper to taste.

Brown meat in a little oil; set aside.

Line baking dish with zucchini slices.

Mix uncreamed cottage cheese with beef and spread over zucchini slices.

Season tomato juice with herbs, salt and pepper and pour over other ingredients.

Top with cheese.

Bake at 375° F. (190° C.) until zucchini squash is tender and cheese blends with other ingredients.

This recipe may be eaten hot as a main course or cold as an appetizer.

MUFFINS, BREAD, AND PANCAKES

Basic Muffin and Bread Recipe

Nuts suitable for this recipe are walnuts, almonds, pecans, and filberts (hazel nuts). Peanuts should not be used. Although they are usually very expensive, some people prefer unroasted raw cashews. Raw cashews are highly perishable so you must be sure that they have been stored properly. Roasted cashews most often contain starch and are, therefore, not permitted. Your choice of nuts should depend upon price, availability, and personal taste preference. Almonds are usually the least expensive and the choice of most people because of their delicate flavor.

Almonds with skins (brownish in color) are suitable for this recipe although, at the beginning of the diet, blanched almonds (without the fibrous skin) will be less gas-forming. After marked improvement, almonds with skins may be used. Twenty-five pounds boxes (or larger) may often be purchased at a discount. If large amounts are bought, they should be kept in the refrigerator or deep freeze to prevent rancidity. In the appendix (page 128), further instructions are given as to how to order the nuts in the most inexpensive way.

The nuts must be ground to a fine consistency—a consistency similar to whole wheat flour. If they are overground, they turn into nut butter which may be used but will make the batter a bit more fluid.

It is advisable to grind your own nuts for the first 3-4 weeks you try the diet. It is true that ground nuts are available and would be a time saver. It is strongly advised, however, that you grind your own so that you can be sure that the ground nuts are fresh and pure with no added extenders. When you have decided to commit yourself to the diet for a longer period, then the ground nuts can be purchased in large quantities in *sealed* boxes.

If the nuts are ground in a blender, do not process more than ¾ cup at one time. Grind to the consistency of whole wheat flour stopping the blender occasionally and scraping around the sides with a kitchen knife or spatula.

The food processor grinds nuts satisfactorily; use the steel blade and make sure it runs long enough to grind the nuts to the consistency of whole wheat flour.

The nuts may also be ground in an electric or manual food grinder.

In the recipes that follow, the term "nut flour" will be used interchangeably with the term "ground nuts"; they mean the same thing.

The following ingredients make 16 muffins.
Preheat oven to 375° F. (190° C.)

2½ cups ground nuts
¼ cup melted butter or
   ¼ cup homemade
   yoghurt, or small amount
   of fruit juice, or pure
   apple butter (add last and
   adjust amount depending
   on the consistency of the
   batter)

½ cup honey† (more or less
   as desired)
1 teaspoon baking soda
1/8 teaspoon salt (optional)
3 eggs (if eggs must be
   avoided, use puréed fruit
   to hold ingredients
   together)

†HONEY: All recipes calling for honey as a sweetener work better if honey is in liquid form. If honey has crystallized, melt over low heat.

Using a blender:
After grinding the nuts in the blender, empty them into a bowl.
Place eggs and honey into blender, and mix thoroughly.
Add the egg mixture to the nuts and blend by hand or with an electric beater.
Add butter or yoghurt as needed to bring to a muffin batter consistency.
Blend in baking soda and salt.

Using a food processor:
After grinding nuts, allow the ground nuts to remain in the processor bowl.
Add other ingredients, adding butter or yoghurt last according to how much liquid you need to bring the batter to a muffin batter consistency.

Line cupcake tins with paper cupcake liners.
Spoon batter into cupcake tins filling about one-half full.
Bake at 375° F. (190° C.) for about 15-20 minutes or until muffins spring back when pressed.
It is difficult to bake "light", high muffins without regular flour and the muffins may fall after they have been removed from the oven. This will not affect their taste.

Variations:
1. Add ⅓ cup raisins or currants.
2. Add juice of one orange and some grated orange rind.
3. Add grated orange rind and chopped dried fruit cut into small pieces. About ½ cup of any of these: apricots, sun dried pineapple, apples, pears.
4. Add 1-2 teaspoons of grated orange rind and ½ teaspoon almond flavor.
5. NUT BREAD - Add one more egg (4 altogether) to batter and bake in a well-buttered, 1-quart baking dish.
6. BANANA NUT BREAD - Add one more egg and two mashed, extra-ripe bananas to batter.
7. COCONUT-NUT MUFFINS - Substitute dried, unsweetened, grated coconut for part of the nut flour. Do not introduce coconut substitution until diarrhea has cleared up.

Cheese Bread

This bread can be sliced and used for French toast; dip in beaten egg and fry in butter.
Syrup of hot honey (with a little water added) may be used to top French toast.
Heat oven to 350° F. (180° C)

2-½ cups ground blanched almonds (or other allowable nut)
¼ cup softened butter
1 cup bland cheese (brick, colby, or mild cheddar)
cut into very small pieces
1 teaspoon baking soda
1/8 teaspoon salt
3 eggs beaten

Mix butter, nut flour, and cheese.
Add eggs, baking soda, and salt.
Pour into a well buttered loaf pan (approx. 4 x 8 inch) and bake until golden brown on top.

Banana Pancakes

1 ripe banana, mashed
1 egg
butter for frying

Beat ingredients together.
Drop on a greased pan and brown over medium heat.
Turn and brown other side.
Serve hot with honey syrup (honey diluted with water and heated)†

†Add maple extract and a little butter to hot honey syrup for a maple syrup substitute.

Zucchini Muffins

3 cups grated zucchini
3 eggs, beaten
3 cups nut flour
⅓ cup melted butter

½-⅔ cup liquid honey (use
less, if desired)
2 teaspoons cinnamon
1 teaspoon baking soda
½ teaspoon salt

Mix almond flour, melted butter, honey, and zucchini.
Add beaten eggs, cinnamon, salt, and baking soda. Mix well.
Bake in muffin tins, lined with papers, at 350° F. (180° C.) for about 20 minutes or until done.

CAKES

Banana Cake

3 cups nut flour
3 eggs, beaten
¼ cup melted butter
½-⅔ cup honey

1 teaspoon baking soda
2 mashed bananas
(extra-ripe)

Mix all ingredients.
Pour into a buttered baking pan.
Bake at 350° F. (180° C.) until top springs back when touched (about 40 minutes).

Carrot Cake

1½ cups nut flour
1½ cups finely shredded
   carrots
¾ cup honey
½ cup raisins
½ cup walnuts (optional)

1 teaspoon baking soda
½ cup butter
2 eggs
1 teaspoon cinnamon
pinch salt
1 teaspoon vanilla

Add honey and eggs to softened butter and blend.
Blend in nut flour, soda, salt, cinnamon, and vanilla.
Add carrots, raisins, and nuts.
Bake at 350° F. (180° C.) for 45-60 minutes.
This cake has a tendency to overflow; therefore, use a large baking pan. A one-quart (1 litre) loaf pan lined with greased waxed paper is satisfactory.
This recipe may be used as a carrot pudding by decreasing the amount of almond flour.

Cheese Cake

The cheese cake filling may be made without a crust but for special occasions, when you want a crust, line the bottom of a small loaf pan with almond honey crisp recipe (see page 94), keeping it as thin as possible.
Bake crust and cool thoroughly.

Filling:

3 eggs
⅓ cup honey
½ cup homemade yoghurt or cream cheese made from yoghurt (see pg.115)

2 cups uncreamed cottage cheese (dry curd)
2 teaspoons vanilla extract
1-2 teaspoons grated lemon rind

Place all ingredients in blender or food processor (metal blade) putting eggs in first so that blender blades will turn freely.
Blend until smooth stopping, if necessary, every 15 seconds to push ingredients down, scraping the sides of the container at the same time with a spatula.
Pour into loaf pan with or without crust.
If desired, place drained, unsweetened canned pineapple slices on top of filling.
Bake in oven at 350° F.(180° C.) for about 30 minutes or until edges are brown.
Cool and refrigerate.

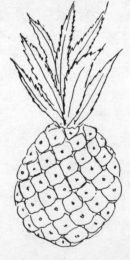

Nut Torte

1½ cups blanched almonds
   or pecans
½ cup honey
8 egg whites

Grind nuts in blender placing only about ¾ cup in blender at one time.
Return ground nuts to blender, add honey, and blend well.
In a large mixing bowl, beat egg whites until stiff.
Very gradually fold honey-nut mixture into egg whites.
Pour into three greased layer cake pans.
Bake at 350° F. (180° C.) for about 35 minutes or until a kitchen knife comes out clean.
Cool.
Fill between layers with custard filling or honey frosting.

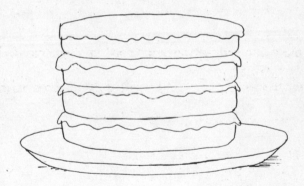

COOKIES

Almond-Honey Crisps

This recipe may also be used to make a piecrust.

1 cup whole almonds   *2 teaspoons vanilla*
¼ cup butter   *(unsweetened)*
⅓-½ cup honey

Process nuts in a blender for only a few seconds until nuts are coarsely chopped. Do not overchop or you will get a flour-like texture which is not suitable for this recipe.
Place chopped almonds in a bowl and set aside.
Put butter, honey, and vanilla in blender, pushing ingredients down to bottom of container before turning blender on.
Process for about 30 seconds until ingredients are whipped.
Transfer mixture to bowl containing chopped nuts and blend thoroughly with a spatula.
Spread in a shallow cake pan and bake at 375° F. (190° C.) until golden brown.
Cut into squares while still warm.

Cheese Cookies

½ cup dry curd cottage cheese   *1 teaspoon honey*
1 egg white   *2 teaspoons nut flour*

Mix ingredients.
Drop on greased cookie sheet.
Bake in 325° F. (160° C.) oven until brown.

Date-Filled Cookies

4 cups nut flour
⅓ cup butter, melted
¼ teaspoon baking soda

¼ teaspoon salt
½ cup honey

Mix all ingredients well.
Roll into small balls.
Place on a greased cookie sheet and press balls into flat cookies with the back of a buttered teaspoon.
Bake at 300° F. (150° C) until golden brown.
Remove from pan and cool.

Filling:
1 lb. pitted dates (California
dates only)
⅓ cup water

Put dates and water in a covered oven-safe saucepan and bake in the oven until soft. This should take about 15 minutes in a 350° F. (180° C.) oven. This date mixture can be cooked on top of stove but it has a tendency to scorch if not stirred constantly.
Stir occasionally while in oven.
Heat in oven until thick.
Cool.
Spread date filling between two cookies.

Monster Cookies

5 cups nut flour
1 cup raisins
1 cup walnut pieces
1 cup flaked unsweetened
   coconut

½ cup melted butter
1 cup honey
2 eggs, beaten
1 teaspoon baking soda
1/8 teaspoon salt

Mix all ingredients.
Drop by large tablespoonfuls onto a greased cookie sheet.
Press flat with a buttered fork. If fork is greased, it will not stick.
Bake at 325° F. (160° C.) until golden brown (15-20 minutes).

Peanut Butter Cookies

½ cup butter
1 cup peanut butter, no
   additives
½ cup honey

2 eggs
¼ teaspoon baking soda
1 teaspoon vanilla

Cream butter until soft.
Add peanut butter and mix thoroughly.
Add remaining ingredients.
Drop on greased cookie sheet and bake in 325° F. (160° C.) oven
for 10 minutes.

Pumpkin Cookies

3 cups nut flour
1 cup mashed, cooked,
 drained pumpkin or fresh
 or frozen winter squash
 such as butternut or
 acorn. Do not use canned
 pumpkin. Summer squash
 such as zucchini is too
 watery for this recipe.

½ cup butter
1 egg
¾ cup honey
1 teaspoon baking soda
¼ teaspoon salt
¼ teaspoon cinnamon
¼ teaspoon nutmeg
1 teaspoon vanilla
1 cup raisins

Mix dry ingredients and raisins. Set aside
Mix egg, butter, honey and vanilla in blender.
Add pumpkin or squash to egg mixture and blend thoroughly.
Add wet ingredients to the dry mixture.
Drop by rounded teaspoonfuls 2 inches apart on lightly greased cookie sheet.
Bake 15 minutes at 375° F. (190° C.) until lightly browned.
Transfer to wire rack to cool.
Makes about 4 dozen cookies.

(Recipe courtesy of Nancy Ferguson)

FROSTINGS

Cream Cheese Frosting

1½ cups dry curd cottage
*   cheese or drained*
*   homemade yoghurt*
honey to sweeten

Place a little liquid honey in blender.
Gradually add dry curd cottage cheese or drained yoghurt.
Blend until smooth.
It may be necessary to stop blender occasionally and press cheese down so that the blender blades can make contact.
Use as a frosting on carrot cake or banana cake.

Honey Frosting

1 cup honey
1 egg white, beaten
1 teaspoon vanilla

Boil the honey until a drop forms a firm ball in cold water.
Add gradually to beaten egg white.
Whip until stiff and add vanilla.
This frosting is marshmallow-like and remains spreadable for hours.
Use as a frosting for cakes; this frosting is especially good on the nut torte.

DESSERTS

Apple Custard Pie

4 or 5 baking apples
1 tablespoon lemon juice
½ cup honey
3 eggs
¾ cup homemade yoghurt
*   or*

homemade French cream
(see pg.118)
¼ cup apple cider
¼ teaspoon nutmeg
2-3 tablespoons chopped
    almonds or walnuts

Core and cut the apples into eighths.
Toss them in lemon juice which has been mixed with honey.
Arrange the apple slices round side down in a pie plate with a circle around the outer edge and another circle inside that, filling in the center.
Bake in oven at 400° F. (200° C.) for 20 minutes.
Beat the eggs slightly, stir in yoghurt or French cream, apple cider and nutmeg.
Pour egg mixture over the apples and continue baking another 10 minutes.
Sprinkle the top with the chopped nuts and bake 10 minutes longer or until the top is golden and the center firm.
Cool on a rack before cutting.

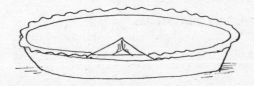

Applesassies

½ *cup butter*   1 cup nut flour
½ *cup honey*   ¼ teaspoon baking soda
2 *eggs, lightly beaten*   1 cup walnuts, chopped
⅔ *cup homemade*   ¾ cup raisins
   applesauce

Melt butter in a double boiler.
Stir in honey, eggs, and applesauce.
Mix baking soda with nut flour and stir into butter mixture.
Stir in raisins and walnuts, saving a few walnut pieces for topping.
Turn into a greased 9 inch square pan.
Sprinkle with the reserved walnuts.
Bake at 350° F. (180° C.) for about 30 minutes.
Cool in pan and serve topped with honey-sweetened whipped uncreamed cottage cheese or French cream.

(Recipe courtesy of Anne Haas Hall)

Baked Honey Apple Slices

½ *cup honey*   2 *teaspoons butter*
juice of 1 lemon   ½ *teaspoon cinnamon*
3 *large cooking apples*

Mix honey and lemon juice in shallow baking dish or pie pan.
Peel and core apples.
Cut apples in quarters, then slices.
Place in honey-juice mixture, coating well.
Dot with butter.
Bake in a moderate oven, 350° F. (180° C.) for about 30-40 minutes or until tender.
Baste with pan liquid twice during baking.
Can be topped with same cheese mixture as Applesassies (above).

Custard

2 eggs
1 cup uncreamed cottage
   cheese (dry curd)
2 teaspoons vanilla extract

8 teaspoons honey
dash of nutmeg
pinch of salt

Beat uncreamed cottage cheese and eggs in blender or food processor until very smooth.
Add honey, vanilla and salt and beat thoroughly.
Pour mixture into custard cups.
Sprinkle nutmeg on top of each cup.
Place custard cups in a pan half filled with water.
Bake at 350° F. (180° C.) for 20 minutes. Increase heat to 375° F. (190° C.) for another ten minutes or until browned on top.

Honey-Glazed Whole Apples

4 medium cooking apples
1 cup water
1 cup honey

½ cup uncreamed cottage
cheese (dry curd) which
has been blended until
smooth with a little
homemade yoghurt

Pare and core apples.
Bring water and honey to a boil in a deep saucepan.
Slowly cook 2 apples at a time in a covered pan in the syrup until apples are tender, turning apples occasionally.
Remove to dessert dishes.
Boil syrup until thick.
Cool syrup slightly and pour over apples.
Serve warm or chilled topped with blended uncreamed cottage cheese or French cream.

Honey-Walnut Baked Apples

large apples for baking   *1 tablespoon honey for each*
raisins   *apple*
walnut pieces   *cinnamon*

Choose a variety of apple that bakes well such as McIntosh, Spy, Ida Red.

Core the apples with a sharp knife leaving them whole.

Arrange apples in a baking dish.

Mix together enough raisins (or currants) and walnuts with honey to fill the cored-out apples.

Add cinnamon to this mixture according to taste.

Fill the apples with honey mixture.

Bake at 350° F. (180° C.) until apples are tender when poked with a fork (about 1 hour).

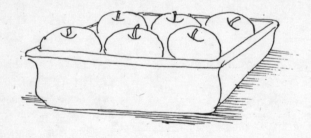

Ice Cream

*1 mashed banana or ½ cup
puréed unsweetened
peaches, pineapple, or
strawberries (small can
of frozen orange juice
may be used instead of
fruit)*

*1-2 cups homemade yoghurt
honey or saccharin for
sweetening according to
taste
1/8 teaspoon salt*

Blend ingredients well.

Place in paper cups or popsicle molds and freeze.

For real ice cream texture, this mixture may be placed in a ice cream maker.

Adjust amounts of ingredients depending upon the volume of your machine.

If you have an ice cream maker which calls for crushed ice, you can avoid having to crush the ice by doing the following:

In the space in which the crushed ice is to be placed, pour 1 cup of cold water.

Measure about 2 cups of ordinary salt and make layers of ice cubes, alternating with salt, until the space is filled. Use all the salt by the time you reach the top.

It is wise to have available plenty of ice cubes; save up the equivalent of about 6 trays before starting.

Pour another cup of cold water around the top of the ice cubes. Start up the motor of the ice cream maker; it should be done in less than an hour.

Variation: Add 1 or 2 raw eggs to the mixture for a creamier texture.

Instant Blender Ice Cream

2 cups homemade yoghurt
1 quart frozen fruit
  (strawberries,
  raspberries, sliced

peaches, blueberries)
Note: Do not thaw fruit!
honey to sweeten

Place ½ cup yoghurt in blender.
Gradually add frozen fruit and the remaining yoghurt alternately.
Add honey to taste.
Blend until thick.
Store in freezer until ready to eat.
This ice cream is thick and smooth and should be eaten soon after making.
If it is refrozen, it will crystallize.

Variation: Freeze yoghurt in ice cube tray and in blender mix the frozen yoghurt cubes with pineapple juice or frozen orange juice (or a mixture of both juices). Use about 6 yoghurt ice cubes and ½ cup juice adding small amounts of juice to obtain a thick consistency.

Lemon Soufflé

1 tablespoon melted butter
½ cup honey
¼ cup almond flour

3 eggs
juice of 1 lemon
1 cup homemade yoghurt

Separate egg whites and beat until stiff.
Beat egg yolks.
Add butter, honey, almond flour, and lemon juice to egg yolks and mix well.
Fold egg whites into mixture.
Pour into greased soufflé dish or deep baking dish.
Set in a pan of water and bake at 350° F. (180° C.) for about 30 minutes.
Soufflé is done when an inserted knife comes out clean.

Orange Mousse

2 cups homemade yoghurt
2 envelopes unflavored
  gelatin
3 eggs, separated
2 oranges (optional)

6 tablespoons frozen orange
  juice concentrate
½ cup honey (more or less
  as desired)

Peel oranges removing as much of the white membrane as possible. Remove seeds and section oranges. Cut each section in half and set aside.

Into top of a double boiler or saucepan put egg yolks which have been beaten well with a fork.

Blend ½ cup of yoghurt and frozen orange juice concentrate with the egg yolks.

If using saucepan, place mixture over low heat and stir until hot.

If using double boiler, place mixture over boiling water and stir until hot. Add honey and stir thoroughly.

Place contents of two envelopes of gelatin in ½ cup cold water for a few minutes to soften.

Add softened gelatin to hot mixture stirring constantly for a few minutes. Remove from heat.

Add enough yoghurt to increase volume of mixture to 3-4 cups and mix thoroughly.

Note: For each envelope of gelatin, do not exceed two cups of mixture. Place in refrigerator until mixture begins to set. This should take about 1 hour.

Beat egg whites until stiff.

Fold orange sections into beaten egg whites.

Fold orange-egg white mixture into gelatin mixture.

Return to refrigerator until gelatinized completely.

Variations: Other fruits may be used: canned, unsweetened crushed pineapple, puréed strawberries, apricots or peaches.

(Recipe courtesy of Nancy Marcellus)

Pineapple Cheese Dessert

1 envelope unflavored
  gelatin
1/8 cup cold water
2 beaten egg yolks
2 stiffly beaten egg whites
½ cup unsweetened crushed
  pineapple

1 teaspoon lemon juice
½ teaspoon lemon rind,
  grated
½ cup uncreamed cottage
  cheese (dry curd)
¼ cup honey
dash of salt

Soften gelatin in cold water.

Combine egg yolks, pineapple, lemon juice, lemon rind, honey, and salt.

Cook over hot water until thick.

Add gelatin and stir until dissolved.

Remove from heat, add cheese.

Chill until set.

Fold in stiffly beaten egg whites.

Spoon into individual molds and return to refrigerator.

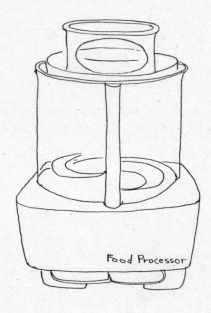

Food Processor

Pumpkin Pie

The almond honey crisp recipe (see pg.94) may be used as a crust or this recipe may be made without a crust and eaten as a custard or pudding.

Filling:

3 eggs, beaten
1 cup homemade yoghurt
or uncreamed cottage
cheese (dry curd) puréed
½ cup honey
2 cups of prepared squash
or pumpkin (canned not
permitted)†

Spices: 2 teaspoons
cinnamon, 1 teaspoon
nutmeg, ½ teaspoon
ground cloves.
Spices may be varied
according to preference.

All ingredients should be mixed thoroughly. This may be done in a large mixing bowl using a beater, or in a blender, or in a food processor. Because of the large volume, it is advised that only part of the ingredients be placed in the processor or blender at one time to avoid overflow.

Pour into a large pie pan or two smaller ones.

Bake at 375°F. (190°C.) or until a knife comes out clean.

May be served warm or cold.

†To prepare squash or pumpkin:

Use winter squash (hubbard, acorn, or butternut).

Remove seeds and steam, boil, or bake until tender.

Scoop out insides discarding skin. Drain.

A large pumpkin may be baked or cooked until tender in the same way as the squash.

Place pumpkin in a bowl and let stand to drain.

Scoop out insides.

Freeze what is not used.

SWEET TREATS, JAM

Candied Nuts

1 lb. nuts (almonds,   2 egg whites
walnuts, pecans,   ½-¾ cup honey depending
hazelnuts) shelled   upon desired sweetness
If hazelnuts are used, rub in   ¼ cup melted butter
towel to remove skins.   pinch of salt
          pinch of cinnamon

Place nuts on large shallow pan and toast in oven at 300° F. (150° C.) for 10 minutes.
Cool.
Beat egg whites with salt until peaks form.
Gradually add honey and continue beating until honey and egg whites are thoroughly mixed.
Fold in nuts and cinnamon.
Coat the large shallow pan with melted butter.
Spread nut and egg white mixture over buttered pan.
Bake in oven at 300° F. (150° C.) for 30 minutes turning nuts every 10 minutes until butter disappears.
Let cool in pan.
Cut or break into bite-size pieces and store in covered container.

(Recipe courtesy of Judy Newman)

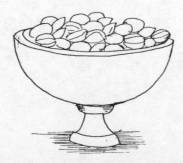

Granola Chews

¼-⅓ *cup butter*
½ *cup honey*
½ *cup raisins*
½ *cup unsweetened,*
   grated coconut

1 *cup coarsely chopped nuts*
   (almonds, pecans, or
   walnuts)
½ *teaspoon salt*

In a saucepan, stir butter and honey over low heat until melted and blended.
Remove from heat and add remaining ingredients, combining well.
Spread mixture in an ungreased square 8 inch baking pan.
Bake at 350° F. (180° C.) for about 25 minutes until set.
Cool, cut in squares.

Quick, Uncooked Coconut Ball Candy

1 *cup liquid honey*
½ *cup unsweetened, grated*
   coconut
½ *cup chopped nuts*

Blend ingredients and roll into balls using buttered hands (to prevent mixture from sticking to hands).
Balls may be rolled in chopped nuts.

Vanilla Candy

½ cup water
1 lb. honey (about 2 cups)
1 teaspoon vinegar

1 teaspoon vanilla extract
   (more, if desired)
2 tablespoons butter
crushed nuts (optional)

Heat honey with vinegar and water in a large pot.
Allow to boil gently until a soft ball forms when dropped into cold water.
Remove from heat and add vanilla extract and butter.
Mix thoroughly with a spoon.
If nuts are to be used, add nuts to honey mixture.
Pour into a flat, buttered **metal** pan and cool.
Place in freezer until hard. Only then can it be cracked into small bite-size pieces.
Remove pan from freezer; place it on a board. Using a clean screw driver as a wedge, crack candy in several places by hitting screw driver handle with a hammer.
Return to freezer to store.
This recipe may be used for making nut logs as follows:
Use 1-2 cups pecan or walnut halves
When honey mixture is ready to remove from heat, add nuts, butter, and vanilla and mix thoroughly.
Cool nut-honey mixture and spoon onto wax paper (doubled in thickness).
Roll into logs and refrigerate.
Slice as needed.

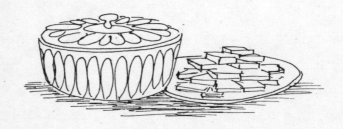

Lolly Pops

Have available small clean sticks; may be purchased in hardware store. Follow the recipe for vanilla candy by heating honey, vinegar and water in a large pot.

Allow to boil gently until a *firm* ball forms when dropped into cold water. Remove from heat and add vanilla extract but *no butter*.

Place sticks about 4 inches apart on a greased cookie sheet and pour approximately 2 tablespoons of hot mixture at the top of each stick allowing mixture to cover about ½ inch of the top of stick.

When the candy has hardened, remove lolly pops and wrap separately.

Variation: Flavorings such as anise or cinnamon may be added with the vanilla.

Becky's Magic Toffee

This recipe is a variation of the vanilla candy recipe.

½ cup water	*1 tablespoon vanilla extract*
1 lb. honey	*1 tablespoon baking soda*
1 teaspoon vinegar	

Heat honey, vinegar, and water in a large pot.

Allow to boil gently until a *firm* ball forms when dropped into cold water. Remove from heat, place pot in sink, add vanilla extract and baking soda.

Stir briskly but only until baking soda is thoroughly blended in and toffee mixture foams up.

When the foaming begins to subside, pour into a well-buttered pan and cool.

When candy is firm enough, it may be cut into bite size pieces using kitchen shears or cracked with a blunt instrument.

Variation: When candy has cooled enough to handle, it can be pulled like taffy and then cut into pieces. Children will enjoy the taffy pull.

(Recipe courtesy of Becky Smith)

JAMS

Jams can be made with many different fruits: strawberries, raspberries, peaches, apricots, black currants, or a combination of these. Commercial pectin is not to be used.

To make jam, add ½ cup honey for each quart of prepared fruit.

Add the smallest amount of water possible to simmer the jam and keep it from sticking and burning at the beginning of cooking.

Stir until ingredients are well blended, then simmer, stirring occasionally to prevent sticking.

As jam becomes thicker, stir more often to prevent scorching.

The jam is done when it becomes thick and forms droplets on the edge of a spoon.

The cooking process should take from 1 - 1½ hours depending on the amount of water to be evaporated.

The jam may not be as thick as ordinary jam. Do not risk scorching it to get it thicker.

Place small amounts in clean containers and freeze. Thaw as needed.

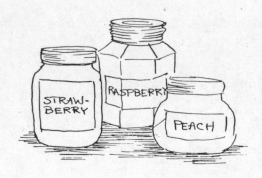

BEVERAGES

Fruit Juice Spritzer
(Replacement for pop)

Combine fruit juice† with Perrier water or club soda and ice to make a nutritious, "fizzy" drink.

†Naturally sweetened juices suitable for this recipe are apple cider, orange, grapefruit, pineapple, and grape.

Milk Shakes

For 1 cup:
  ½ cup homemade yoghurt   *peaches, raspberries,*
  ½ cup fresh or frozen fruit   *bananas, blueberries.†*
  such as stawberries,

Place yoghurt in blender and then add fruit.
Sweeten to taste with a little honey or saccharin.
Blend until thick and creamy.

†If fresh fruit is used, add a few ice cubes to chill drink.

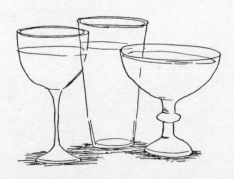

Party Punch†

1 large can unsweetened pineapple juice

1 large can frozen orange juice and 1 can water

Mix juices in punch bowl, add ice cubes.
Float fruit slices or berries on top.

†Keep a bowl of punch available, especially in warm weather, to avoid the temptation of beverages that are not permitted. Make sure punch bowl is sturdy.

Piña Colada

unsweetened canned pineapple juice

ice cubes

Fill blender no more than half full with unsweetened pineapple juice.
Add no more than 4 or 5 ice cubes†
Run blender for about 45 seconds until drink is frothy and creamy.
Serve at once.

†If sherbet is desired, rather than a drink, add about 10 ice cubes.

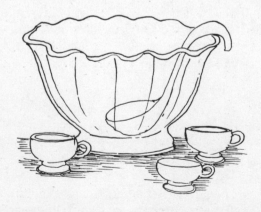

MILK PREPARATIONS AND INFANT FORMULA

YOGHURT

Yoghurt is one of the oldest foods known to man. Wherever people milked cows, goats, mares, sheep, or camels, a product similar to yoghurt was eaten. Kefir, Kumiss, fermented acidophilus milk, and Bulgarian milk are all similar to yoghurt, differing only in the kinds of microbes introduced into the milk.

If milk is left unrefrigerated in a warm environment, many types of microbes (bacteria and yeast) in the air, as well as some remaining in the milk, even after Pasteurization, start multiplying and using the milk sugar, lactose, as a source of energy. The result is soured milk which often has a bitter, unpleasant taste and consistency. In making yoghurt, this process is controlled by getting rid of the mixture of microbes and introducing only those which produce the tart and tasty product you desire.

You may use powdered, skimmed, 2%, or whole milk. If you use powdered milk, add only the amount of powder which you would use to make regular fluid milk. **Do not** add additional milk powder to fluid milk in order to get a thicker yoghurt or more protein as you will not get a "true" yoghurt and **it will be detrimental** to those on the Specific Carbohydrate Diet.

Whole milk makes a very tasty yoghurt but if you are eliminating fat for a particular reason, you may use low fat milk. If you do, you must be careful while heating as it scorches more readily than whole milk.

INSTRUCTIONS
1. Bring one quart (or liter) milk to the simmer stage and remove from heat. Stir often to prevent scorching and sticking to the bottom of the pan.
2. Cover and cool until it has reached room temperature or below (may be placed in refrigerator to hasten cooling). It is very important that

you allow the temperature to drop sufficiently or you will kill the
bacterial culture you are now ready to introduce.

3. Remove about one-half cup cooled milk and make a paste with one-
   quarter cup of a good quality commercial yoghurt. The commercial
   yoghurt you use should be unflavored and unsweetened. Buy one
   that contains only milk or milk solids and bacterial culture, if possible.
   It is usually unnecessary to buy yoghurt culture separately since
   commercial yoghurt is very satisfactory to use as a ''starter''. If
   you find it impossible to buy commerical yoghurt which contains
   only milk and bacterial culture, then you are advised to buy yoghurt
   culture (''starter'') separately. After removing what is needed, return
   the container of commercial yoghurt to the coldest part of the
   refrigerator for use as a starter for the next batch of homemade
   yoghurt.

   Saving some yoghurt from a previous batch of homemade yoghurt
   to use to start a new batch is not as satisfactory as using commercial
   yoghurt as a ''starter'' each time since the manufacturers of
   commercial yoghurt make every effort to use ''lively'' bacterial
   strains and extremely large numbers of bacteria in the manufacturing
   process. The conditions of home refrigeration most often do not
   promote the survival of yoghurt bacteria to the same degree as do
   the conditions maintained by the commercial producers of yoghurt.
   Homemade yoghurt, made by using some from the last batch as
   a ''starter'', often fails to solidify (coagulate) properly due to
   insufficient live bacteria to properly convert the milk sugar.

4. Mix the paste with the remainder of the cooled milk and stir
   thoroughly.

5. Pour milk into any appropriate sized container, cover, and let stand
   for at least 24 hours at 100°-110° F. (38-43° C.). (If you forget
   to remove it after 24 hours, and the fermentation goes on longer,
   all the better.) Under no circumstances should the fermentation time
   be decreased to less than 24 hours. This fermentation time
   should supersede any other instructions which may accompany a
   commercial yoghurt maker.

   The source of heat used during the 24-hour fermentation is critical.
   It is very important to get the temperature correct at 100-110° F.
   (38-43° C.) before you proceed with the fermentation. Too high
   a temperature will kill the bacterial culture and will prevent the proper

"digestion" (conversion) of the lactose. Too low a temperature will prevent activation of bacterial enzymes and will result in incomplete "digestion" of the lactose.

A thermos-type of yoghurt maker may **not** be satisfactory for this long fermentation period inasmuch as the hot water surrounding the thermos will not stay warm. The electric commercial yoghurt makers control the temperature perfectly but the amount of yoghurt that can be made at one time is limited. The ideal source of heat is a large electric warming tray. If it has a temperature-regulating dial, use a thermometer to set the dial properly (a mouth thermometer is satisfactory). If the warming tray does not have a dial to control the temperature, cover the surface of the tray with a thickness of metal (such as a metal cake rack) or **fire-resistant** material (such as a teflon-treated ironing board cover) and allow the tray to remain on for about five minutes before placing the thermometer on the surface to determine the temperature. If too warm, use a thicker piece of metal or material. By using the large surface of the electric warming tray, a gallon of yoghurt can be made at one time in two (plastic or ceramic) ½ gallon containers. An electric crock pot (set to low) or a heating pad, both checked for temperature, may be used.

Some people use their ovens; the pilot in a gas oven usually keeps the temperature in the oven within the correct range. If using the oven of an electric stove, change the oven light to a 60-watt bulb. Turning on the oven light (with a 60-watt bulb) should create enough warmth to make yoghurt; always check the temperature with a thermometer first. Sometimes the oven door must be propped ajar with a little stick to achieve the correct temperature range.

Caution: Upon completion of yoghurt fermentation, replace regular oven bulb.

6. Allow the yoghurt to remain on the heat for a minimum of 24 hours to insure that all lactose is completely "digested". Remove from heat gently and refrigerate.

    While this yoghurt may not be as thick as commercial yoghurt, it will be a **true** yoghurt since virtually all of the lactose has been digested by the bacterial culture and further lactose digestion will not be required by intestinal cells.

Cream Cheese

1 Line a colander with a clean cloth (a dish towel is satisfactory).
2. Place colander on a bowl.
3. Pour chilled yoghurt into lined colander and allow to drain for about 6-8 hours (need not be refrigerated while draining).
4. Lift cloth by two opposite ends, place on flat surface, and with a spatula, scrape "cream cheese" off and refrigerate. It will be quite tart; a little liquid honey may be worked in with a spatula to sweeten.

French Cream

2 cups cream (table cream, half-and-half, or heavy cream)

½ cup commercial yoghurt (see yoghurt recipe for type to use)

Bring cream to simmer stage stirring often as it heats.
Cool cream and follow recipe for homemade yoghurt.
Allow cream to ferment for 24-48 hours.
Refrigerate.
For a creamy rich ice cream, use in ice cream recipe instead of yoghurt or use part yoghurt and part French cream. May also be used as a topping for desserts.

INFANT FORMULA - DISACCHARIDE FREE

This formula may be used for short periods of time until the physician can prescribe a formula which contains no disaccharides. Some commercial formulas which are recommended for diarrhea contain considerable amounts of corn syrup (containing maltose and isomaltose). As a result, some babies with severe diarrhea do not recover when they are used.[1] Check newer formulations as they appear on the commercial market to ensure that they are disaccharide-free.

The following formula (about 2 cups) contains approximately 90 mg calcium, 175 mg phosphorous, 72 mg potassium, 0.40 mg iron, 17 gm protein, 0.3 gm fat, and 2.7 gm carbohydrate.

Babies one year and younger need approximately 500-700 mg calcium per day. An additional source of calcium would, therefore, be necessary if this formula is used more than a few days. Please discuss this with your physician.

The following ingredients should be used and enough water added to bring the total up to about 2 cups (17 fluid oz or 500 ml).

3 tablespoons uncreamed cottage cheese (dry curd) (1.2 oz or 33 gm)

1 tablespoon unrefined safflower oil (0.7 fluid oz or 19 ml)

It is preferable to purchase the oil already bottled. Health food stores and some large supermarkets usually carry this item. Please read the label carefully and make sure that there is no BHT or BHA added. Addition of vitamin E, beta carotene, or vitamin A is all right.

2 tablespoons pasteurized honey (0.9 fluid oz or 25 ml)

Prior to the preparation of the formula, place the honey and approximately 1 cup of the water in a pressure cooker and heat keeping the honey-water mixture under pressure for 10 minutes. This is to sterilize the honey and kill any microorganisms which cannot be killed by ordinary heat.

Place the dry curds in a blender with the oil.

Blend until very smooth.

Slowly add the honey-water mixture and blend until smooth.

Bring total up to approximately 2 cups (17 fluid oz or 500 ml) with water.

Place in a nursing bottle and make the hole in the nipple slightly larger.

This recipe may be doubled or tripled depending upon how much the baby needs. Keep the unused portions refrigerated and covered. Use within 24 hours after preparation.

The formula contains the following:

Total protein, mainly casein	1.1%
Total carbohydrate	5.0%
Total fat	3.8%

These proportions are comparable to breast milk with the exception of the carbohydrate. Breast milk contains 2% more carbohydrate. However, the formula does not contain all the vitamins and minerals that are needed daily by the baby. The formula may be tried, with your doctor's concurrence, for a limited period for constipation or diarrhea. When the condition is alleviated, return to the normal formula.

1. Fisher, S.E., G. Leone, R.H. Kelly. 1981. Chronic protracted diarrhea: Intolerance to dietary glucose polymers. Pediatrics 67:271-273.

GLOSSARY

Carbohydrates	various types of sugar, starch, and dietary fibers
Digestion	(1) the process of reducing large food molecules into simpler compounds and, thereby, making it possible for them to be absorbed from the digestive tract into the bloodstream (2) splitting food molecules
Disaccharides	sugars composed of two parts (two molecules) chemically linked and which require digestion before they can be absorbed into the bloodstream
Disaccharidases	a group of enzymes embedded within the membranes of the intestinal absorptive cells. These enzymes (lactase, sucrase, maltase, and isomaltase) digest (split) the double sugars lactose, sucrose, maltose, and isomaltose respectively
Enteropathy	an intestinal disease
Enzymes	chemical compounds, made by cells, which are responsible for chemical reactions carried on by those cells
Fermentation	the chemical breakdown of carbohydrates (sugars, starch, and fiber) by intestinal microbes resulting in the production of hydrogen gas, carbon dioxide gas, and various other products such as lactic acid, acetic acid and alcohol.
Fructose (levulose)	(1) a monosaccharide sugar found in honey and fruits (2) one of the monosaccharide sugars released, along with glucose, when sucrose is digested (3) a "predigested" sugar
Flora	various bacteria, yeast, and other microscopic forms of life in the intestinal contents
Galactose	a monosaccharide sugar released, along with glucose, when the milk sugar, lactose, is digested

Glucose *(dextrose)*	(1) a single sugar (see monosaccharides) found in sources such as fruits and honey (2) a single sugar released, along with fructose, when sucrose is digested (3) a single sugar released, along with galactose, when lactose is digested (4) the single sugars released when maltose and isomaltose are digested (5) the type of sugar making up the starch molecule; starch is a chain of glucose molecules
Lactase	an enzyme embedded within the membranes of intestinal cells (within the microvilli) which digests (splits) lactose into glucose and galactose
Lactose	(1) milk sugar (2) a disaccharide sugar composed of one part glucose and one part galactose chemically linked
Lumen	interior space of intestine
Maltase	an enzyme embedded within the membranes of intestinal cells (within the microvilli) which digests (splits) maltose into two molecules of glucose
Isomaltase	an enzyme embedded within the membranes of intestinal cells (within the microvilli) which digests (splits) isomaltose into two molecules of glucose
Maltose	a disaccharide sugar composed of two molecules of glucose chemically linked; most of the maltose found in the intestinal tract is derived from starch which has undergone partial digestion
Isomaltose	a disaccharide sugar composed of two molecules of glucose chemically linked differently than maltose; most of the isomaltose found in the intestinal tract is derived from starch which has undergone partial digestion
Molecule	a substance containing two or more atoms. Example: water is a molecule which contains two atoms of hydrogen and one atom of oxygen (H_2O).
Monosaccharides	(1) single sugars including glucose, fructose, and galactose which require no further digestion in order to be absorbed into the bloodstream (2) "predigested" sugars
Mucosa *(intestinal)*	the lining of the intestinal tract which is formed by the the intestinal cells and which comes in contact with the contents of the intestinal tract

Peristalsis	involuntary waves of muscular contraction and relaxation which propel the contents of the intestine forward
Polysaccharides	a class of carbohydrates consisting of many chemically linked sugar molecules; starch is the most familiar example
Putrefaction	the chemical breakdown of proteins by intestinal microbes resulting in the formation of ammonia and other substances
Refined Carbohydrate	a carbohydrate such as cornstarch or white sugar which has been separated from substances with which it is normally associated in the natural or whole state. Refined carbohydrates usually have their calories left intact but have lost most, if not all, of the fiber, vitamins, and minerals found in the whole foods from which they have been extracted.
Starch	(1) a long chain of glucose molecules chemically linked to each other (2) one of the carbohydrates found throughout the plant kingdom; grains and potatoes contain large amounts of starch (3) a polysaccharide
Sucrose	(1) a disaccharide sugar composed of one part glucose and one part fructose chemically linked (2) ordinary table sugar extracted from sugar cane or sugar beets
Sucrase	an enzyme embedded within the membranes of the intestinal cells (within the microvilli) which digests (splits) sucrose into glucose and fructose
Sugars	chemical compounds of varying sweetness which include fructose, glucose, isomaltose, lactose, maltose, and sucrose
Villi	fingerlike projections (forming hills and valleys) which normally make up the absorptive surface of the small intestine; they become flattened in various conditions
Microvilli	fingerlike projections normally present on *individual* intestinal absorptive cells; normally, digestive enzymes are embedded within microvilli but, in many conditions, microvilli disappear along with their digestive enzymes
Vitamins	substances present in small amounts in natural foodstuffs (or supplements) which are essential for cellular function and the lack of which in the diet results in disease. The cells, with minor exceptions, cannot make vitamins.

Herb's Bean Pancakes

1   cup cooked and well drained white beans
1   small onion
1   egg
⅛ teaspoon baking soda
salt to taste
homemade yoghurt as needed

A food processor, blender or electric mixer may be used. If using a blender, place egg in blender first so that blades can turn easily. Place all ingredients in bowl or blender and blend until batter is smooth.

If batter is not a consistency which can be poured easily (as for pancakes), add yoghurt, a teaspoon at a time, and blend in well. Using a well-buttered frying pan, pour batter as you would pancake butter.

Using medium heat, turn pancakes after about 8 - 10 minutes. Cook an additional 8 minutes on other side.

The above ingredients make 4 medium-sized pancakes.

Do not use beans that have not been drained well as batter will be too watery.

A large batch of beans can be prepared in advance and can be frozen in suitably sized containers.

APPENDIX

CHEESES

Permitted cheeses are those which contain virtually no lactose. In order for a cheese to be free of lactose, the manufacturing process must include separation and removal of the whey (containing most of the lactose) from the curd as well as a "curing" of the remaining lactose by the addition of a bacterial culture.

Cheeses Permitted	Cheeses Not Permitted
Use those in italics freely; the others occasionally	Cottage Cheese (regular)
Asiago	Cream
Blue	Feta
Brick	Gjetost
Brie	Gruyere
Camembert	Mozzarella (Pizza cheese)
Cheddar, mild, medium, or sharp	Neufchatel
Colby	Primost
Edam	Ricotta
Gorgonzola	Processed cheese slices or spreads
Gouda	
Havarti	
Limburger	
Monterey (Jack)	
Muenster	
Parmesan (if already grated, check to make sure that there are no added milk solids)	
Port du Salut	
Roquefort	
Romano	
Stilton	
Swiss	
Uncreamed cottage cheese (dry curd)	

Amount of Sucrose Commonly Added to Foods

Food category	Average percent by weight
Baked goods, baking mixes	11.42
Breakfast cereals	26.71
Grain products, such as pastas or rice dishes	1.43
Processed cheeses	24.56
Frozen dairy desserts	9.31
Processed fruits, juices and drinks	12.58
Fruit ices, water ices	12.38
Processed meat products	2.87
Processed vegetables, juices	13.25
Condiments, relishes, salt substitutes	26.82
Soft candies	44.74
Jams, jellies, sweet spreads	32.72
Sweet sauces, toppings, syrups	30.96
Gelatin, puddings, fillings	19.11
Processed nut products	8.14
Gravies, sauces	5.66
Hard candy	49.98
Chewing gum	42.30
Granulated sugar	97.92
Instant coffee and tea	12.60
Baby Products	
Cereals	2.55
Formulas	4.76
Processed fruit	12.25
Meat products	0.44
Poultry products	0.58
Processed vegetables	2.89
Puddings	12.09
Soups, soup mixes	0.36

Sources for Vitamin Supplements

It is important to find vitamin supplements which contain no sugar, starch, wheat, soy, whey, or yeast. A yeast-based supplement is not permissible while on this diet. This eliminates brewer's yeast and most natural B-complex vitamins.

People living near large cities or towns should be able to contact companies or individuals who can supply them with information about the fillers and binders used in various vitamin preparations. The information given on pages 42 and 43 of this book gives the reader some idea as to what strengths of each vitamin are appropriate.

Although it is more convenient to obtain vitamins locally, often this is not possible. In these cases, the author suggests that you write to the Freeda Vitamin Company, 36 East 41st St., New York City, N.Y. 10017 for a catalogue and price list. Their Quin B Strong (without zinc) is the recommended B-Complex vitamin for people on the Specific Carbohydrate Diet. Cut the tablets in quarters or halves depending upon the amount needed. In Chapter 7, amounts are suggested for members of the B-Complex vitamin family which are believed to be suitable for the average adult or child who has a malabsorption problem. Since these vitamins are not scored for cutting, it will take a little patience to cut them evenly. Do not be too concerned if you find you cannot be exact.

If sending to this company for your vitamins, you should estimate the amount of return postage and include this with your money order so that there will be minimum delay. The company will follow up with a statement and will credit you with any overpayment.

If you have a credit card, ask Freeda if you may use it and in this way avoid all the time-consuming details of obtaining money orders, figuring out the currency exchange rate and guessing what the postage will be. Freeda's toll free number is 1-800-777-3737.

There are many companies making good quality B-Complex vitamins but it is beyond the scope of this book to investigate them. If you prefer dealing with a company in your vicinity, it is your responsibility to write to them and ask about the forbidden binders and fillers such as starch, lactose, whey powder, and sucrose which are often combined with vitamin compounds. If you take vitamins with starch and other forbidden carbohydrates, you lose the benefit of the diet.

SOURCES FOR GROUND AND WHOLE NUTS

For the first three weeks that you try the diet, it is advisable that you buy nuts by the pound (or kilo) and grind them yourself. People in or near large cities, with a little effort, can locate a source of nuts at a reasonable price. You have a choice of health food stores, bulk food stores, wholesale/retail outlets (listed in phone book), and specialty companies which supply food items for those on special diets. Bakeries use nuts in their baked goods; ask at the bakery about their supplier. You might want to call the Almond Board of California (415-495-6420) or the California Independent Almond Growers (209-667-4855) to help you locate a reasonably priced supplier.

When you are convinced, after the first 3-4 weeks, that the diet is helping you, then it is wise to order the ground (minced), blanched almonds or ground pecans in a large quantity. There should be a considerable saving when you order in a 25 lb. or 35 lb. box. It is important to keep the ground nuts under refrigeration or in a freezer to prevent rancidity.

People living in outlying areas may have to order nuts through the mail. It is suggested that you inquire at your local bakery (bakeries use lots of nuts), health or bulk food store as to where the nearest source of supply is located. It may be an importer in a large town nearby. Those living in the eastern parts of North America may find that pecan farms in Georgia are a convenient and reasonably priced source. Those living in the middle west and the west will probably find walnut and almond farms in California, British Columbia, Oklahoma, etc. that are willing to ship directly to the customer. Be sure to check into the mailing or freight charges before ordering. These charges can often exceed the cost of the nuts.

The Juice Dilemma

During 1991, a leading commercial juice manufacturer had been found guilty of mislabeling their fruit juices. Their labels stated that there was no sugar, corn syrup, or sweetener added, but it was found that this labeling was deceptive. There have been many incidents like this in the past relating to fruit juice labeling. This is unfortunate because some companies are reliable but it is beyond the scope of this book to check them all out. We have requested and received letters from Welch's and Dole's relating to two of their products and we feel that we can safely recommend Welch's purple grape juice in the jar and Dole's unsweetened pineapple juice in the can. These may be used in addition to apple cider (not apple juice) from a local cider mill (after you have talked to the owner) and juices that you squeeze yourself. We realize that there are many juice companies who are honest in their labeling and we suggest that, should you want to use any of them, you do your own detective work by calling and asking for a letter to back up statements on their labels, specifically, that no sweeteners have been added.

Dry Cottage Cheese

It has been stated on page 38 that you should try to find a source of dry cottage cheese. In most provinces in Canada, Beatrice Foods manufactures and distributes this product. It comes in 250 gram containers. If your grocer does not normally carry it, ask the manager to order you a case of 12 containers. If you ask for less, the store may be reluctant to get it. This cheese freezes well and you can freeze the case taking it out as you need it and thawing it overnight or placing the container in the microwave for 2 minutes. In other areas, you can inquire at health food stores, delicatessens, or farmer's markets in an effort to find dry cottage cheese.

REFERENCES

Chapter 1: Past and Present

1. Haas, S.V. and M.P.Haas. 1951. *Management of Celiac Disease*. J.B. Lippincott Co., Philadelphia.
2. Dohan, F.C. 1966. Cereals and schizophrenia - data and hypotheses. Acta Psychiatry Scandanavia 42:125-152.
3. Dohan, F.C. 1978. Schizophrenia: Are some food-derived polypeptides pathogenic? In *The Biological Basis of Schizophrenia*. Eds. G. Hemmings and W.A. Hemmings. University Park Press, Baltimore.
4. Worthen, D.B. and J.R. Lorimer. 1979. *Enteral Hyperalimentation with Chemically Defined Elemental Diets: A Source Book*, 2nd ed. Norwich-Eaton Pharmaceuticals, Norwich, New York.
5. Russell, R.I. 1981. *Elemental Diets*. CRC Press, Florida.
6. Morin, C.L., M. Roulet, C.C. Roy, and A. Weber. 1980. Continuous elemental enteral alimentation in children with Crohn's disease and growth failure. Gastroenterology 79:1205-1210.
7. Sandberg, D.H., P.M. Tocci, and R.M. McKey. 1974. Decrease in sweat sodium chloride concentrations on limited diets. Pediatric Research 8:386.

Chapter 2: Scientific Evidence Relating to Diet

1. Haas, S.V. and M.P. Haas. 1951. *Management of Celiac Disease*. J. B. Lippincott Co., Philadelphia.
2. deDombal, F.T. 1968. Ulcerative colitis: definition, historical background, etiology, diagnosis, natural history and local complications. Postgraduate Medical Journal 44:684-692.
3. Herter, C. 1908. *On Infantilism from Chronic Intestinal Infection*. MacMillan, New York.
4. Herter, C. 1910. Observations on intestinal infantilism. Transactions of the Association of American Physicians 25:528.
5. Gee, S. 1888. On the coeliac affliction. St. Bartholomew's Hosptial Report 24:17.
6. Cozzetto, F.J. 1963. Intestinal lactase deficiency in a patient with cystic fibrosis. Report of a case with enzyme assay. Pediatrics 32:228-233.
7. Jones, R.H.T. 1964. Disaccharide intolerance and mucoviscidosis. Lancet 2:120-121.

8. Donaldson, R.M.,Jr. and J.D. Grybsoki. 1973. Carbohydrate intolerance. In *Gastrointestinal Disease*. Eds. M.H. Sleisenger and J.S. Fordtran. W.B. Saunders Co., Philadelphia.

9. Sandberg, D.H., P.M. Tocci, and R.M. McKey. 1974. Decrease in sweat sodium chloride concentrations on limited diets. Pediatric Research 8:386.

10. Struthers, J.E.,Jr., J.W.Singleton, and F. Kern,Jr. 1965. Intestinal lactase deficiency in ulcerative colitis and regional ileitis. Annals of Internal Medicine 63:221-228.

11. Wright, R., and S.C. Truelove. 1965. A controlled therapeutic trial of various diets in ulcerative colitis. British Medical Journal 2:138-141.

12. Cady, A.B., J.B. Rhodes, A. Littman, and R.K. Crane. 1967. Significance of lactase deficit in ulcerative colitis. Journal of Laboratory and Clinical Medicine 70:279-286.

13. Kirschner, B.S., M.V. DeFavaro, and W. Jensen. 1981. Lactose malabsorption in children and adolescents with inflammatory bowel disease. Gastroenterology 81:829-832.

14. Truelove, S.C. 1961. Ulcerative colitis provoked by milk. British Medical Journal 1:154-160.

15. McMichael, H.B., J. Webb, and A.M. Dawson. 1965. Lactase deficiency in adults: A cause of "functional" diarrhoea. Lancet I:717-720.

16. Chalfin, D. and P.R. Holt. 1967. Lactase deficiency in ulcerative colitis, regional enteritis and viral hepatitis. American Journal of Digestive Diseases 12:81-87.

17. Gudmand-Hoyer, E. and S. Jarnum. 1970. Incidence and clinical significance of lactose malabsorption in ulcerative colitis and Crohn's disease. Gut 11:338-343.

18. Tandon, R., H. Mandell, H.M. Spiro, and W.R.,Thayer. 1971. Lactose intolerance in Jewish patients with ulcerative colitis. American Journal of Digestive Diseases 16:845-848.

19. VonBrandes, J.W., and H. Lorenz-Meyer. 1981. Diet excluding refined sugar: a new perspective for the treatment of Crohn's disease? A randomized controlled study. Z. Gastroenterologie 19:1-12.

20. Alun Jones, A., E. Workman, A.H. Freeman, R.J. Dickinson, A.J. Wilson, and J.O. Hunger. 1985. Crohn's disease: Maintenance of remission by diet. Lancet II:177-180.

21. Morin, C.L., M. Roulet, C.C. Roy, and A. Weber. 1980. Continuous elemental enteral alimentation in children with Crohn's disease and growth failure. Gastroenterology 79:1205-1210.

22. VanEys, J. 1977. Nutritional therapy in children with cancer. Cancer Research 37:2457-2461.

23. Poley, J.R. 1984. Ultrastructural topography of small bowel mucosa in chronic diarrhea in infants and children: Investigations with the scanning electron microscope. In *Chronic Diarrhea in Children*. Ed. E. Lebenthal. Nestlé, Vevey/Raven Press, New York.

24. Salyers, A.A. 1979. Energy sources of major intestinal fermentative anaerobes. American Journal of Clinical Nutrition 32:158-163.
25. McCarrison, R. 1922. Faulty food in relation to gastrointestinal disorders. JAMA 78:1-8.

Chapter 3: Intestinal Microbes: The Unseen World

1. Bengson, M.H. 1979. Effects of bioisolation on the intestinal microflora. American Journal of Clinical Nutrition 23:1525-1532.
2. Kopeloff, N. 1930. *Man Versus Microbes*. Garden City Publishing Co.,Inc., Garden City, New York.
3. Haenel, H. 1970. Human normal and abnormal gastrointestinal flora. American Journal of Clinical Nutrition 23:1433-1439.
4. Shahani, K.M. and A.D. Ayebo. 1980. Role of dietary lactobacilli in gastrointestinal microecology. American Journal of Clinical Nutrition 33:2448-2457.
5. Simon, G.L. and S.L. Gorbach. 1981. Intestinal flora in health and disease. In *Physiology of the Gastrointestinal Tract*, Vol.2. Ed. L.R. Johnson. Raven Press, New York.
6. Feibusch, J.M. and P.R. Holt. 1982. Impaired absorptive capacity for carbohydrate in the aging human. Digestive Diseases and Sciences 27:1095-1100.
7. Gracey, M.S. 1981. Nutrition, bacteria and the gut. British Medical Bulletin 37:71-75.
8. McEvoy, A., J. Dutton, and O.F.W.James. 1983. Bacterial contamination of the small intestine is an important cause of occult malabsorption in the elderly. British Medical Journal 287:789-793.
9. Dubos, R. 1962. *The Unseen World*. The Rockefeller Institute Press, New York.
10. Pope, C.II. 1983. Involvement of the esophagus by infections, systemic illnesses and physical agents. In *Gastrointestinal Disease*. Eds. M.H. Sleisenger and J.S. Fordtran. W. B. Saunders Co., Philadelphia.
11. Rolfe, R.D. and S.M. Finegold. 1980. Inhibitory interactions between normal fecal flora and Clostridium difficile. American Journal of Clinical Nutrition 33:2539.
12. Donaldson, R.M. 1964. Normal bacterial populations of the intestine and their relation to intestinal function. The New England Journal of Medicine 270:938-945.
13. King, C.E. and P.E. Toskes. 1979. Small intestine bacterial overgrowth. Gastroenterology 76:1035-1055.
14. Haas, S.V. and M.P. Haas. 1951. *Management of Celiac Disease*. J.B. Lippincott Co., Philadelphia.
15. Flexner, S. and J.E. Sweet. 1906. The pathogenesis of experimental colitis and the relation of colitis in animals and man. Journal of Experimental Medicine 8:514-535.

16. Morgan, H.D. 1907. Upon the bacteriology of the summer diarrhea of infants. British Medical Journal 2:16-19.

17. Bassler, A. 1922. Treatment of cases of ulcerative colitis. Medical Record 101:227-229.

18. Bargen, J.A. 1924. Experimental studies on etiology of chronic ulcerative colitis. JAMA 83:332-336.

19. Crohn, B.B., L. Ginzburg, and G.D. Oppenheimer. 1932. Regional ileitis. JAMA 99:1323-1329.

20. Menon, T.B. 1930. The pathology of chronic colitis in the tropics. Indian Journal of Medical Research 18:137-141.

21. Bargen, J.A., M.C. Copeland, L.A. Buie. 1931. The relation of dysentery bacilli to chronic ulcerative colitis. Practitioner 127:235-247.

22. Hurst, A.F. 1931. Ulcerative colitis. Proceedings of the Royal Society of Medicine 24:785-803.

23. Felsen, J. and W. Wolarsky. 1953. Acute and chronic bacillary dysentery and chronic ulcerative colitis. JAMA 153:1069-1072.

24. Takeuchi, A., S.B. Formal, and H. Sprinz. 1968. Acute colitis in Rhesus monkey following peroral infection with Shigella flexneri. American Journal of Pathology 52:503-529.

25. Staley, T.E., L.D. Corley, and E.W. Jones. 1970. Early pathogenesis of colitis in neonatal pigs monocontaminated with Escherichia coli. Fine structural changes in the colonic epithelium. American Journal of Digestive Diseases 15:923-935.

26. DuPont, H.I., S.B. Formal, R.B. Hornick, M.J. Snyder, J.P. Libonati, D.G. Sheahan, E.H. LaBrec, and J.P. Kalas. 1971. Pathogenesis of Escherichia coli diarrhea. The New England Journal of Medicine 285:1-9.

27. Metchnikoff, E. 1908. The Prolongation of Life. G.P. Putnam's Sons, New York.

28. Robins-Browne, R.M. and M.M. Levine. 1981. The fate of ingested lactobacilli in the proximal small intestine. American Journal of Clinical Nutrition 34:514-519.

29. Kolars, J.C. M.D. Levitt, M.M. Aouji, and D.A. Savaino. 1984. Yoghurt - an autodigesting source of lactose. New England Journal of Medicine 310:1-3.

30. McCarrison, R. 1922. Faulty food in relation to gastrointestinal disorders. JAMA 78:1-8.

31. Necheles, H. and C. Beck. 1965. Lactobacillus and intestinal flora. Applied Therapeutics 7:463-465.

32. Sandine, W.E., K.S. Muralidhara, P.R. Elliker, and D.C. England. 1972. Lactic acid bacteria in food and health. Journal of Milk and Food Technology 35:691-702.

33. Johnson, W.C. 1974. Oral elemental diet. Archives of Surgery 108:32-34.

34. George, W.L., R.D. Rolfe, V.L. Sutter, and S.M. Finegold. 1979. Diarrhea and colitis associated with antimicrobial therapy in man and animals. American Journal of Clinical Nutrition 32:251-257.

35. Willoughby, J.M.T. 1982. The alimentary system. In *Iatrogenic Diseases*, 2nd ed. Eds. P.P. D'Arcy and J.P. Griffin. Oxford University Press, New York.

36. Ziv, G.M., M.J. Paape, and A.M. Dulin. 1983. Influence of antibiotics and intramammary antibiotic products on phagocytosis of Staphylococcus aureaus by bovine leukocytes. American Journal of Veterinary Research 44:385-388.

37. Low-Beer, T.S. and A.E. Reed. 1971. Progress report. Diarrhoea: Mechanisms and treatment. Gut 12:1021-1036.

38. Keusch, G.T., and D.H. Present. 1976. Summary of a workshop on clindamycin colitis. Journal of Infectious Diseases 133:578-587.

39. Toffler, R.B., E.G. Pingoud, and M.I. Burrell. 1978. Acute colitis related to penicillin and penicillin derivatives. Lancet 2:707-709.

40. Sakurai, Y., H. Tsuchiya, F. Ikegami, T. Funatomi, S. Takasu, and T. Uchikoshi. 1979. Acute right-sided hemorrhagic colitis associated with oral administration of ampicillin. Digestive Diseases and Sciences 24:910-915.

41. Boriello, S.P., R.H. Jones, and I. Phillips. 1980. Rifampicin-associated pseudomembranous colitis. British Medical Journal 281:1180-1181.

42. Fournier, G., J. Orgiazzi, B. Lenoir, and M. Dechavannne. Pseudomembranous colitis probably due to rifampicin. Lancet I:101.

43. Friedman, R.J., I.E. Mayer, J.T. Galambos, and T. Hersh. 1980. Oxacillin-induced pseudomembranous colitis. American Journal of Gastroenterology 72:445-447.

44. Saginur, R., C.R. Hawley, and J.G. Bartlett. 1980. Colitis-associated metronidazole therapy. Journal of Infectious Disease 141:772-774.

45. Thomson, G., A.H. Clark, K. Hare, and W.G.S. Spilg. 1981. Pseudomembranous colitis after treatment with metronidazole. British Medical Journal 282:864-865.

46. Weidema, W.F., M.F. Von Meyenfeidt, P.B. Soeters, R.I.C. Wesdorp, and J.M. Greep. 1980. Pseudomembranous colitis after whole gut irrigation with neomycin and erythromycin base. British Journal of Surgery 67:895-896.

47. Coleman, D.L. P.H. Juergensen, M.H. Brand, and F.O. Finkelstein. 1981. Antibiotic-associated diarrhoea during administration of intraperitoneal cephalothin. Lancet 1:1004.

48. Lishman, A.H., I.J. Al-Jumaili, and C.O.Record. 1981. Spectrum of antibiotic-associated diarrhoea. Gut 22:34-37.

49. Taylor, A.G. 1976. Toxins and the genesis of specific lesions: Enterotoxin and exfoliatin. In *Mechanisms in Bacterial Toxinology*. Ed. A.W. Bernheimer. John Wiley and Sons, New York.

50. Arbuthnott, J.P. and C.J. Smith. 1979. Bacterial adhesion in host/pathogen interactions in animals. In *Adhesion of Microorganisms to Surfaces*. Eds. D.C. Ellwood and J. Melling. Academic Press, London.

51. Salyers, A.A. 1979. Energy sources of major intestinal fermentative anaerobes. American Journal of Clinical Nutrition 32:158-163.

52. Moore, W.E.C. and L.V. Holdeman. 1975. Discussion of current bacteriological investigations of the relationships between intestinal flora, diet, and colon cancer. Cancer Research 35:3418-3420.

Chapter 4: Breaking the Vicious Cycle

1. Stephen, A.M. 1985. Effect of food on the intestinal microflora. In *Food and the Gut*. Eds. J.O. Hunter and V.A. Jones. Bailliére Tindall, London.
2. Weijers, H.A. and J.H. vandeKamer. 1965. Treatment of malabsorption of carbohydrates. Modern Treatment 2:378-390.
3. Oh, M.S., K.R. Phelps, M.Traube, J.L. Barbosa-Salvidar, C. Boxhill, and H.J. Carroll. 1979. D-Lactic acidosis in a man with the short-bowel syndrome. New England Journal of Medicine 301:249-252.
4. Stolberg, L., R. Rolfe, N. Gitlin, J. Merritt, L. Mann, J. Linder, and S. Finegold. 1982. D-Lactic acidosis due to abnormal gut flora. New England Journal of Medicine 306:1344-1348.
5. Traube, M., J. Bock, and J.L. Boyer. 1982. D-Lactic acidosis after jejunoileal bypass. New England Journal of Medicine 307:1027.
6. Lifshitz, F. 1982. Necrotizing enterocolitis and feedings. In *Pediatric Nutrition*. Ed. F. Lifshitz. Marcel Dekker, Inc., New York.
7. Jonas, A., P.R. Flanagan, and G.C. Forstner. 1977. Pathogenesis of mucosal injury in the blind loop syndrome. Journal of Clinical Investigation 60:1321-1330.
8. Lee, P.C. 1984. Transient carbohydrate malabsorption and intolerance in diarrheal diseases of infancy. In *Chronic Diarrhea in Children*. Ed. E. Lebenthal. Nestlé, Vevey/Raven Press, New York.
9. Johnson, W.C. 1974. Oral elemental diet. Archives of Surgery 108:32-34.
10. Jarnum, S. 1976. Chemically defined diets in medicine. Nutrition and Metabolism 20 (Supplement 1):19-26.

Chapter 5: Carbohydrate Digestion

1. Go, V.L.W. and W.H.J. Summerskill. 1971. Digestion, maldigestion, and the gastrointestinal hormones. American Journal of Clinical Nutrition. 24:160-167.
2. Gee, S. 1888. On the coeliac affliction. St. Bartholomew Hospital Report 24:17.
3. Moog, F. 1981. The lining of the small intestine. Scientific American 245:154-176.
4. Poley, J. R. 1984. Ultrastructural topography of small bowel mucosa in chronic diarrhea in infants and children: Investigations with the scanning electron microscope. In *Chronic Diarrhea in Children*. Ed. E. Lebenthal. Nestlé, Vevey/Raven Press, New York.

5. Plotkin, G.R. and K.J. Isselbacher. 1964. Secondary disaccharidase deficiency in adult celiac disease (non tropical sprue) and other malabsorption states. New England Journal of Medicine. 271:1033-1037.
6. Burke, V., K.R. Kerry, and C.M. Anderson. 1965. The relationship of dietary lactose to refractory diarrhea in infancy. Australian Paediatric Journal 1:147-160.
7. Kojecky, Z. and Z. Matlocha. 1965. Quantitative differences of intestinal disaccharidase activity following the resection of stomach. Gastroenterologia (Basel) 104:343-351.
8. McMichael, H.B., J. Webb, and A.M. Dawson. 1965. Lactase deficiency in adults: a cause of functional diarrhoea. Lancet 1:717:720.
9. Weser, E. and M.H. Sleisenger. 1965. Lactosuria and lactase deficiency in adult celiac disease. Gastroenterology 48:571-578.
10. Weser, E., W. Rubin, L. Ross, and M.H. Sleisenger. 1965. Lactase deficiency in patients with the "irritable-colon syndrome." New England Journal of Medicine 273:1070-1075.
11. Welsh, J.D., O.M. Zschiesche, J. Anderson, and A. Walker. 1969. Intestinal disaccharidase activity in celiac sprue (gluten-sensitive enteropathy). Archives of Internal Medicine 123:33-38.
12. Prinsloo, J.G., W. Wittmann, H. Kruger, E. Freier. 1971. Lactose absorption and mucosal disaccharidases in convalescent pellagra and kwashiorkor children. Archives of Diseases of Childhood 46:474-478.
13. King, E. and P.P. Toskes. 1979. Small intestine bacterial overgrowth. Gastroenterology 76:1035-1055.
14. Gray, G. 1982. Intestinal disaccharidase deficiencies and glucose-galactose malabsorption. In *The Metabolic Basis of Inherited Disease*. Eds. J.B.Stanbury, J.B.Wyngaarden, D.S.Fredrickson, J.S.Goldstein, and M.S.Brown. 5th ed. McGraw-Hill Book Co., New York.
15. Campos, J.V.M., U.F. Neto, F.R.S. Patricio, J. Wehba, A.A. Carvalho, and M. Shiner. 1979. Jejunal mucosa in marasmic children. Clinical, pathological, and fine structural evaluation of the effect of protein-energy malnutrition and environmental contamination. American Journal of Clinical Nutrition. 32:1575-1591.
16. Brunser, O. and M. Araya. 1984. Damage and repair of small intestinal mucosa in acute and chronic diarrhea. In *Chronic Diarrhea in Children*. Ed. E. Lebenthal. Nestlé Vevey/Raven Press, New York.
17. Dvorak, A.M., A.B. Connell, and G. R. Dickersin. 1979. Crohn's disease: A scanning electron microscopic study. Human Pathology 10:165-177.
18. Lee, P.C. 2984. Transient carbohydrate malabsorption and intolerance in diarrhea disease of infancy. In *Chronic Diarrhea of Children*. Ed. E. Lebenthal. Nestlé, Vevey/Raven Press, New York.
19. Pope, C.E. II. 1983. Involvement of the esophagus by infections, systemic illnesses and physical agents. In *Gastrointestinal Disease*. Eds. M.H. Sleisenger and J.S. Fordtran. W. B. Saunders Co., Philadelphia.

20. Anderson, I.H., A.S. Levine, and M.D. Levitt. 1981. Incomplete absorption of the carbohydrate in all-purpose wheat flour. New England Journal of Medicine 304:891-892.

21. Feibusch, J.M. and P.R. Holt. 1982. Impaired absorptive capacity for carbohydrate in the aging human. Digestive diseases and Sciences 27:1095-1100.

22. Rackis, J.J. 1975. Oligosaccharides of food legumes: Alpha-galactosidase activity and the flatus problem. In *Physiological Effects of Food Carbohydrates*. Eds. A. Jeanes and J. Hodge. American Chemical Society, Washington, D.C.

23. Fisher, S.E., G. Leone, R.H. Kelly. 1981. Chronic protracted diarrhea: Intolerance to dietary glucose polymers. Pediatrics 67:271-273.

24. Lebenthal, E., L. Heitlinger, P.C. Lee, K.S. Nord, C. Holdge, S.P. Brooks, and D. George. 1983. Corn syrup sugars: In vitro and in vivo digestibility and clinical tolerance in acute diarrhea of infancy. Journal of Pediatrics 103:29-34.

25. Juliano, B.O. 1972. Physicochemical properties of starch and protein in relation to grain quality and nutritional value of rice. Internation Rice Research Institute (Los Banos) Annual Report.

26. Weiner, M. and J. VanEys. 1983. In *Nicotinic Acid*. Marcel Dekker, Inc. New York.

27. Cooke, W.T. and G.K.T. Holmes. 1984. *Coeliac Disease*. Churchill Livingstone, New York.

28. Gunja-Smith, Z., J.J. Marshall, C. Mercier, E.E. Smith, and W.J. Whelan. 1970. A revision of the Meyer-Bernfield model of glycogen and amylopectin. FEBS Letters 12:101-104.

29. Davidson, G.P. and R.R.W. Townley. 1977. Structural and functional abnormalities of the small intestine due to nutritional folic acid deficiency in infancy. Journal of Paediatrics 90:590-595.

Chapter 6: Beyond Gluten

1. Dicke, W.K. 1950. Coeliakie, een onderzoek naar de nadelige invloed van sommige graansoorten op de lijder ann coeliakie. Thesis, Utrecht.

2. Matthews, D.M. 1975. Intestinal absorption of peptides. Physiological Review 55:537-608.

3. Moog, F. 1981. The lining of the small intestine. Scientific American 245:154-176.

4. Haas, S.V. and M.P. Haas. 1951. *Management of Celiac Disease*. J.B. Lippincott Co., Philadelphia.

5. Cluysenaer, O.J.J. and J.H.M.vanTongeren. 1977. *Malabsorption in Coeliac Sprue*. Martinus Nijhoff Medical Division, Hague.

6. Bleumink, E. 1974. Allergens and toxic protein in food. In *Coeliac Disease*. Eds. W.T.J.M. Hekkens and A.S. Peña. Stenfert Kroese, Leiden.

7. Weiser, M.M. 1976. An alternative mechanism for gluten toxicity in coeliac disease. Lancet 1:567-569.

8. Baker, P.G. and A.E. Read. 1976. Oats and barley toxicity in coeliac patients. Postgraduate Medical Journal 52:264-268.

9. Strunk, R.C., J.L. Pinnas, T.J. John, R.C. Hansen, and J.L. Blazovich. 1978. Rice hypersensitivity associated with serum complement depression. Clinical Allergy 8:51-58.

10. Vitoria, J.C., C. Camarero, A. Sojo, A. Ruiz, and J. Rodriguez-Soriano. 1982. Enteropathy related to fish, rice and chicken. Archives of Disease in Childhood 57:44-48.

11. Phelan, J.J., F.M.Stevens, W.F. Cleere, B. McNicholl, C.F. McCarthy, and P.F. Fottrell. 1978. The detoxification of gliadin by the enzymic cleavage of a side-chain substituent. In *Perspectives in Coeliac Disease*. Eds. B. McNicholl, C.F. McCarthy and P.F. Fottrell. University Park Press, Baltimore.

12. Stevens, F.M., J.J. Phelan, B. McNicholl, F.R. Comerford, P.F. Fottrell, and C.F. McCarthy. 1978. Clinical demonstration of the reduction of gliadin toxicity by enzymic cleavage of side-chain substituent. In *Perspectives in Coeliac Disease*. Eds. B. McNicholl, C.F. McCarthy, and P.F. Fottrell. University Park Press, Baltimore.

13. Cooke, W.T. and G.K.T. Holmes. 1984. *Coeliac Disease*. Churchill Livingstone, New York.

14. Congdon, P., M.K. Mason, S.Smith, A. Crollick, A. Steel, and J. Littlewood. 1981. Small bowel mucosa in asymptomatic children with celiac disease. American Journal of Diseases in Children 135:118-122.

15. Gryboski, J. 1981. False security of a gluten-free diet. American Journal of Diseases in Children 135:110-112.

16. Rubin, C.E., L.L. Brandborg, A.L. Flick, P.Phelps, C. Parmentier, and S. van Niel. 1962. Studies of celiac sprue. III The effect of repeated wheat instillation into the proximal ileum of patients on a gluten free diet. Gastroenterology 43:621-641.

17. Creamer, B. 1966. Coeliac thoughts. Gut 7:569-571.

18. Poley, J.R. 1984. Ultrastructural topography of small bowel mucosa in chronic diarrhea in infants and children: Investigations with the scanning electron microscope. In *Chronic Diarrhea in Children*. Ed. E. Lebenthal. Nestlé, Vevey/Raven Press, New York.

19. King, C.E. and P.P. Toskes. 1979. Small intestine bacterial overgrowth. Gastroenterology 76:1035-1055.

20. Araya, M. and J.A. Walker-Smith. 1975. Specificity of ultrastructural changes of small intestinal epithelium in early childhood. Archives of Disease in Childhood 50:844-855.

21. Brunser, O. and M. Araya. 1984. Damage and repair of small intestinal mucosa in acute and chronic diarrhea. In *Chronic Diarrhea in Children*. Ed. E. Lebenthal. Nestlé Vevey/Raven Press, New York.

22. Holmes, G.K.T., P.L. Stokes, T.M. Sorahan, P. Prior, J.A.H. Waterhouse, and W.T. Cooke. 1976. Coeliac disease, gluten free diet, and malignancy. Gut 17:612-619.

23. Lifshitz, F. and G. Holman. 1966. Familial celiac disease with intestinal disaccharidase deficiencies. American Journal of Digestive Diseases 11:377-387.

24. Berg, N.O., A. Dahlqvist, T. Lindberg, and A. Norden. 1970. Intestinal dipeptidases and disaccharidases in celiac disease in adults. Gastroenterology 59:575-582.

25. Plotkin, G.R. and K.J. Isselbacher. 1964. Secondary disaccharidase deficiency in adult celiac disease (non tropical sprue) and other malabsorption states. New England Journal of Medicine 271:1033-1037.

26. Townley, R.R.W., K.T. Khaw, and H. Schwachman. 1965. Quantitative assay of disaccharidase activities of small intestinal mucosal biopsy specimens in infancy and childhood. Pediatrics 36:911-921.

27. Arthur, A.B. 1966. Intestinal disaccharidase deficiency in children with celiac disease. Archives of Diseases in Children 41:519-524.

28. Littman, A. and J.B. Hammond. 1965. Diarrhoea in adults caused by deficiency in intestinal disaccharidases. Gastroenterology 48:237-249.

29. Anderson, I.H., A.S. Levine, and M.D. Levitt. 1981. Incomplete absorption of the carbohydrate in all purpose wheat flour. New England Journal of Medicine 304:891-892.

Chapter 7: Introducing the Diet

1. Haas, S.V. and M.P. Haas. 1951. *Management of Celiac Disease*. J.B. Lippincott Co., Philadelphia.

2. Kraybill, H.F. 1977. Nonoccupational environmental cancer. In *Advances in Modern Toxicology*. Vol. 3. John Wiley & Sons, New York.

3. Delmont, J. 1983. Milk consumption and rejection throughout the world. In *Milk Intolerance and Rejection*. Ed. J. Delmont. Karger, Basel.

4. Van Soest, P.J. 1981. Some factors influencing the ecology of gut fermentation in man. In *Banbury Report 7 - Gastrointestinal Cancer: Endogenous Factors*. Eds. W.R. Bruce, P. Correa, M. Lipkin, S.R.Tannenbaum, and T.D. Wilkins. Cold Spring Harbor Laboratory.

5. Connon, J.J. and K.N. Jeejeebhoy. 1985. General approach to acute and chronic diarrhea. In *Gastrointestinal Diseases*. Ed. K.N. Jeejeebhoy. Medical Examination Publishing Co., Inc., New Hyde Park, New York.

INDEX

Not all food items have been listed in the index. For a complete listing of permitted foods, see Chapter 8.

ORDER FORM

FOOD AND THE GUT REACTION

	TOTAL TO ENCLOSE
CANADA	
_____ Price per book	$16.95
For orders shipped by 4th class, add $3.50 per book plus $.50 for each additional book	3.50
GST 7% (Tax)	1.43
	$21.88

Note: Non-Canadian orders, deduct $1.43 from total.

Payments by check or money order.

Complete the following:

Send your order to:

THE KIRKTON PRESS
R.R. 1 Kirkton, Ontario
CANADA N0K 1K0
519-229-6795

$ _____ Total price per volume
(including handling, shipping and tax)

X _____ Number of volumes ordered

$ _____ TOTAL ENCLOSED

Name: _____

Address: _____

City, State or Province and Postal Code _____

ORDER FORM

FOOD AND THE GUT REACTION

	TOTAL TO ENCLOSE
CANADA	
_____ Price per book	$16.95
.For orders shipped by 4th class, add $3.50 per book plus $.50 for each additional book	3.50
GST 7% (Tax)	1.43
	$21.88

Note: Non-Canadian orders, deduct $1.43 from total.

Payments by check or money order.

_____

Complete the following:

Send your order to:

THE KIRKTON PRESS
R.R. 1 Kirkton, Ontario
CANADA N0K 1K0
519-229-6795

$ _____ Total price per volume
(including handling, shipping and tax)

X _____ Number of volumes ordered

$ _____ TOTAL ENCLOSED

Name: _____

Address: _____

City, State or Province and Postal Code _____